UNFUCK YOUR KINK

Using Science to Enjoy Mind-Blowing BDSM, Fetishes, Fantasy, Porn, and Whatever Your Pervy Heart Desires

Dr. Faith G. Harper, LPC-S, ACS, A

Microcosm Publishing

Portland, Ore | Cleveland, Ohio

T0300701

UNFUCK YOUR KINK: Using Science to Enjoy Mind-Blowing BDSM, Fetishes, Fantasy, Porn, and Whatever Your Pervy Heart Desires

© Dr. Faith G. Harper, 2024

First edition - 3,000 copies - January 16, 2024

ISBN 9781648413285

This is Microcosm #503

Edited by Olivia Rollins
Cover and design by Joe Biel
This edition © Microcosm Publishing, 2024
For a catalog, write or visit:
Microcosm Publishing
2752 N Williams Ave.
Portland, OR 97227

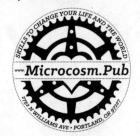

www.Microcosm.Pub/Kink

To join the ranks of high-class stores that feature Microcosm titles, talk to your rep: In the U.S. **COMO** (Atlantic), **ABRAHAM** (Midwest), **BOB BARNETT** (Texas, Arkansas, Oklahoma, Louisiana), **IMPRINT** (Pacific), **TURNAROUND** (Europe), **UTP/ MANDA** (Canada), **NEWSOUTH** (Australia/New Zealand), **GPG** in Latin America, Africa, the Middle East, India, and Asia, or **FAIRE** and **EMERALD** in the gift trade.

Did you know that you can buy our books directly from us at sliding scale rates? Support a small, independent publisher and pay less than Amazon's price at **www.Microcosm.Pub**.

Global labor conditions are bad, and our roots in industrial Cleveland in the '70s and '80s made us appreciate the need to treat workers right. Therefore, our books are MADE IN THE USA.

A version of some of the content in this book was originally published in other works by Dr. Harper. These include *Unfuck Your Intimacy*, *BDSM FAQ*, *Unfuck Your Consent*, *Unfuck Your Blow Jobs*, and *Unfuck Your Cunnilingus*, as well as articles written for various other publications, such as *Out in SA*.

Library of Congress Cataloging-in-Publication Data
    Names: Harper, Faith G., author.
    Title: Unfuck your kink : using science to enjoy mind-blowing BDSM,
      fetishes, fantasy, porn, and whatever your pervy heart desires / Faith
      G. Harper.
    Description: [Portland, OR] : Microcosm Publishing, [2024] | Summary:
      "Tackles the whys, whats, and how-tos of the very wide range of human
      erotic experience, while debunking myths, explaining the science behind
      why we like what we like, and discussing how to engage safely,
      shamelessly, and satisfyingly in BDSM, pornography, fantasies,
      role-play, and fetishes both common and rare. Let the sex positivity
      resound!"-- Provided by publisher.
    Identifiers: LCCN 2023032853 | ISBN 9781648413285 (trade paperback)
    Subjects: LCSH: Fetishism (Sexual behavior) | Sexual dominance and
      submission. | Sex (Psychology)
    Classification: LCC HQ79 .H347 2024 | DDC 306.77/7--dc23/eng/20230830
    LC record available at https://lccn.loc.gov/2023032853

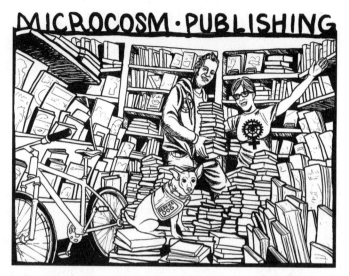

Microcosm Publishing is Portland's most diversified publishing house and distributor, with a focus on the colorful, authentic, and empowering. Our books and zines have put your power in your hands since 1996, equipping readers to make positive changes in their lives and in the world around them. Microcosm emphasizes skill-building, showing hidden histories, and fostering creativity through challenging conventional publishing wisdom with books and bookettes about DIY skills, food, bicycling, gender, self-care, and social justice. What was once a distro and record label started by Joe Biel in a drafty bedroom was determined to be *Publishers Weekly*'s fastest-growing publisher of 2022 and #3 in 2023, and is now among the oldest independent publishing houses in Portland, OR, and Cleveland, OH. We are a politically moderate, centrist publisher in a world that has inched to the right for the past 80 years.

TABLE OF CONTENTS

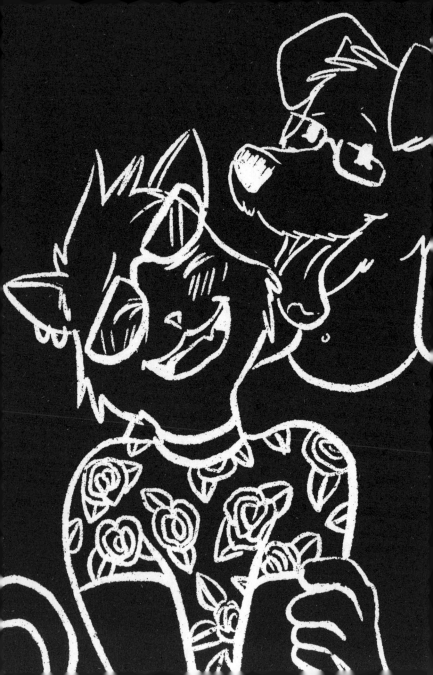

INTRODUCTION: WHAT IS KINK, ANYWAY? AND IS IT BAD? (SPOILER ALERT: NO)

*W*hile a solid portion of people are entirely squicked out by sex, most humans have *something* that gets them off. And if you live in today's world, there's a good chance that you've been told by someone (probably a lot of someones) that you're fucked up and dirty and broken for liking what you like. And I wouldn't have a job if people would just leave people the fuck alone, so here we go with me doing my job:

> **There is nothing wrong with your sexual inclinations, either vanilla or covered in perv sprinkles. There is nothing wrong with consenting adults doing stuff to their own or each other's bodies for the purpose of sexual enjoyment. You are allowed to like what you like.**

Of course, many sexologists for many decades have been saying the same thing. We write, we speak, we do interpretive dance expressing this as a fundamental-fucking-truth. However, the pearl-clutching cultural overlords (who, btw, don't even know what a kinkster's version of a pearl necklace is) continue to challenge our work in order to suppress human autonomy and bodily enjoyment. From the Nazis burning all of Magnus

Hirschfeld's work on sexology in 1933[1] to today's weirdo coomers and their stupid NoFap bullshit.

So this book is going to call that kink-shaming bullshit out. Once again, we're going to go through all the research demonstrating that we are right and the cultural overlords are wrong. And of course, just to spite them, we're going to have some fun along the way.

Since I will always be a sex educator at heart, that journey is going to start out with a bit of background info. In case you haven't noticed, the world of kink has its own vocabulary, so we're gonna get granular about what all these words flying around even mean. Then we're going to get into the science of human sexuality, and the utter normalcy of being who we are. We'll dig into how to communicate about what gets you off, and how to even figure out what you like in the first place. And of course, we'll talk about engaging in practices safely (whether vanilla af or rainbow sprinkles for days . . . safety is always important). Then, finally, I'm also going to answer a bunch of the questions that came flying in when we announced that this book was in the making, cuz y'all asked some great questions!

Now, this is a book about kink, and there are some topics that are sometimes associated with kink (usually by the same aforementioned cultural overloads) that we won't be covering in any great detail. These include being minor-attracted, engaging in acts of pedophilia, and engaging in acts of non-consensual violent activity toward adults (such as sexual assault). These are incredibly complicated and important topics with lots of

---

1 Twenty-fucking-thousand books. And that school district in Texas that's banning books like it's cool? That was the district my kids grew up and attended school in. Sometimes the irony is just too on the nose, enit?

subtleties around the differences between attraction and offense. We will bump into these topics when we talk about the DSM (*The Diagnostic and Statistical Manual of Mental Disorders*), fantasy, and legal considerations, because it would be dishonest to pretend that kink and real violence don't end up categorized in similar ways. But there will be no deep dives into topics that move us out of the kink domain and belong in an entirely different book.

What Do These Words Even Mean?

You've probably seen some kink-related words thrown around all over the place without a clear idea of what they actually mean, and how they interrelate. And if you are new to my books, this is a good place to provide a fair warning that I am a recovering academic who still can't help but insist that we define all terms before we put them into action.

So now you will know what they all mean, too. But try not to pull the "but, actually . . ." card with your friends when they get this stuff wrong . . . just save your knowledge for bar trivia night. And the "ok, but WHY" part of this discussion will come along a bit later in the book. We're just starting with the operational stuff.

Kink

Kink is an umbrella term that references any sexual behaviors that are considered different from our cultural standard of "normal." That standard can be set by the larger culture, or a smaller one. So even something that might be considered pretty normal or benign if you polled all the people who live in the country, like role-playing naughty nurse and grateful patient with a partner or whatever, may seem bizarre, harmful, or even sinful to the individuals who belong to a conservative church in a rural area. A lot of behaviors and preferences that aren't readily categorized end up falling under the kink umbrella as well. The most commonly engaged-in and known-about kink is BDSM (which stands for bondage, domination, sadism, and masochism). But others you may have heard about include furries (the chillest, funnest people ever), role-play (like dressing up as a naughty nurse or a firefighter or whatever), voyeurism (including cucking, which is when someone watches their partner have sex with someone else), and the like. You know Rule 34 of the internet, which states that if something exists there is porn of it? In an even more general sense, if something exists, humans have found a way to make it sexual. Cuz we do that.

Fetish

Fetishes fall under the kink umbrella in that they are also "nontraditional" sexual interests. The term *fetish* is used to describe erotic connection to things that are not (on the surface) considered erotic. Like non-genital body parts (being super into feet is a common fetish we will discuss more later in this book) and inanimate objects generally considered non-sexual (shoes, if we want to stay on the subject of feet). Additionally, certain non-sexual behaviors may also become a necessary part of someone's sex life. Like maybe someone only gets turned on after running on the treadmill and getting really sweaty and grimy. If they don't do that part first, they can't get turned on, even though that behavior isn't foreplay. That would be a fetish too.

No matter the object or behavior in question, though . . . the big differentiation for your bar trivia night is that a fetish is a necessary component of someone's ability to experience sexual satisfaction, whereas a kink isn't a nonnegotiable requirement. Wearing leather gladiator boots to the sex club might be a fun kinky activity for some people, but someone who experiences attraction to shoes as a fetish (retifism) must have engagement with shoes in order to complete their sexual response cycle (which we'll talk about in Chapter 1).

Paraphilia

Ok, now we're getting into more clinical terms. But this is an important one, in that it will help create the framework for many of the other discussions in this book. Paraphilias are typically defined as abnormal sexual desires, especially those that involve activities that are extreme or dangerous. In the past, paraphilias were referred to as "sexual perversions" or "sexual deviancy," which are just other ways of saying hella fun at parties, but we digress.

Historically, the practice of psychology was framed around the idea that anything outside the surrounding cultural norms (in this case we're talking about post-war industrialized Western culture) was a mental illness. Horatio Storer labeled women who liked sex and masturbation as nymphomaniacs. Albert Ellis encouraged women to de-gayify men by fondling them (didn't work, if you were wondering).

We're better than that now. Not always on an individual basis, but at least in regards to the diagnostic criteria we are supposed to follow before deciding if something is a problem or not. The authors of the DSM (which is published by the American Psychiatric Association and contains the official diagnostic criteria for psychiatric disorders of all kinds) still use the term *paraphilia* to refer, clinically, to any non-vanilla sexual interests, noting that having a paraphilia isn't a problem in and of itself. The DSM gets itself involved when a paraphilia becomes what it terms a *paraphilic disorder*. Clinically, a paraphilic disorder is any kink or fetish that is creating problems in life-domain functioning. Someone might try to call a paraphilia a "disorder" just because they consider it deviant, but the American Psychiatric Association says, essentially, "No, sorry . . . deviant based on society standards maybe, but if you aren't hurting anyone or anything and you're just a little sexual weirdo, then go forth and do your sexual weirdo shit . . . it's not a mental illness to want to fill a kiddie pool with mayo and get your rocks off, or whatever."

Now, if you were missing work because you couldn't stand to leave the mayo swim, that would be a problem. Or if you were stealing mayo to fill your pool because you couldn't afford your habit anymore. And yes, even if you think your behavior is weird and abnormal and it's messing with your head. Whatever. *It's only a problem if it is creating actual problems.*

The DSM-5-TR (the current edition at the time of this writing) only contains eight specific paraphilic disorders, all of which require that the issue be ongoing (six months AT LEAST) for it to be considered diagnosable. Why only eight? First of all, anything can become sexualized, so there wouldn't be any way to catch them all like Pokémon.[2] Secondly, the authors of the DSM state that they were focusing on the most common ones. The thirdly point will become apparent as you keep reading. Below, I've included a paraphrased version of the DSM's definitions of these eight specific disorders, along with two less-specific ones. You will notice I've used italics

2 And yes, of course, a Pokémon fetish exists too. In fact, it is common enough that a couple of the Pokémon books published in the original Japanese pay homage to the practice. This writing was scrapped from the English versions.

to emphasize some of the terminology used by the authors of the DSM. This is my own stylistic choice, not one copied over from the DSM. You will notice a theme in what I choose to italicize, which will be important to the rest of our discussions in this book.

Voyeuristic Disorder (302.82 [F 65.3]): Wherein someone experiences recurrent and intense sexual arousal from watching *unsuspecting* people who are engaging in sexual activities or getting dressed/undressed without their knowledge and consent.

Exhibitionistic Disorder (302.4 [F 65.2]): Wherein someone experiences recurrent and intense sexual arousal from the exposure of their genitals to an *unsuspecting* person.

Frotteuristic Disorder (302.89 [F 65.81]): Wherein someone experiences recurrent and intense sexual arousal from touching or rubbing against a *non-consenting* person.

Sexual Masochism Disorder (302.83 [F 65.51]): Wherein someone experiences recurrent and intense sexual arousal from the experience of being humiliated, beaten, bound, or otherwise made to suffer and this arousal manifests as urges, fantasies, or behaviors that are causing *clinically significant distress* or *impairment* in life domains.

Sexual Sadism Disorder (302.84 [F65.52]): Wherein someone experiences recurrent and intense sexual arousal from the physiological or psychological *suffering* of another person and they have acted on these urges with a *non-consenting* person or the urges are causing *clinically significant distress* or *impairment* in life domains.

Pedophilic Disorder (302.2 [F 65.4]): Wherein someone experiences recurrent and intense arousal around the idea of sexual activity with a prepubescent child or children (generally ages 13 or younger). The individual has either *acted* on these urges or the urges are causing *marked distress or interpersonal difficulty*. The individual in question is *at least 16 years old and at least five years older than the child or children referenced*. And the DSM does specifically state that an individual in late adolescence involved in an *ongoing* sexual relationship with a 12- or 13-year-old does not qualify for this diagnosis.

Fetishistic Disorder (302.81 [F 65.0]): Wherein someone experiences recurrent and intense sexual arousal from either the use of non-living objects (like an ironing board or whatever) or a highly specific focus on non-genital body parts (like someone's eyebrows or whatever) and fantasies, urges, and behaviors around these specific attractions are causing *significant distress* or *impairment* in life functioning.

Transvestic Disorder (302.3 [F 65.1]): Wherein someone experiences recurrent and intense sexual arousal from cross-dressing and fantasies, urges, and behaviors around these specific attractions are causing *significant distress* or *impairment* in life functioning. This diagnosis does require specifying whether there is fetishism involved (meaning the arousal comes from the garments themselves) or autogynephilia (meaning the arousal comes from the thoughts or images of oneself as a different gender from the one assigned at birth). The DSM authors point out that the former is more likely related to a fetishistic disorder and the latter may be an indicator of gender dysphoria. The authors also emphasize that this diagnosis only applies if the purpose of the cross-dressing is sexual excitement. This means that when one engages in the behavior it is always or almost always a sexually fulfilling activity, not one that provides a sense of comfort, authenticity, or gender euphoria, or one intended as a statement on gender norms (e.g., dressing as an intentional genderfuck).

Other Specified Paraphilic Disorder (302.89 [F 65.89]): This is a catchall category for other possible paraphilias that are causing a *level of harm* to the individual experiencing these desires or the *non-consenting* living beings that are on the receiving end of these desires. The distress and impairment must be present and clinically significant. And the issue in question must be documented as part of the assigned diagnosis. The DSM authors note some of the common paraphilias that may get diagnosed here, such as zoophilia (sexual attraction to animals), scatologia (sexual pleasure derived from using obscene language), necrophilia (sexual attraction to corpses), coprophilia (sexual pleasure derived from thoughts of or use of feces), klismaphilia (sexual pleasure derived from enemas), or urophilia (sexual pleasure derived from thoughts of or use of urine). All of which have components that could become dangerous, if only because of possible bacteria causing unintended illness.

Unspecified Paraphilic Disorder (302.9 [F 65.9]): This diagnosis is used much like the previous one, except without the specific labeling of the issue. There may not be enough information to know exactly what the issue is, or it may be that the individual is subthreshold for one of the other paraphilia diagnoses but is starting to demonstrate signs of *distress or impairment* that have resulted in them seeking treatment.

Did you notice the pattern in what I chose to italicize? All of these are classified as disorders because they have the potential to cause harm to others (e.g., they involve doing things to non-consenting individuals) or because they cause significant distress or impairment for the sufferer. That's the third reason why there are only eight specified paraphilic disorders and the two general categories are highly specific about what is required to diagnose: if it doesn't cause harm, distress, or impairment, it's not a disorder.

So this clinical stuff is not the fun part. And, to reiterate, chances are you are just a regular perv, not someone living with a paraphilic disorder. But it is important to cover them, because humans do love a good moral panic, and you may bump into these terms (if you haven't already) due to your own proclivities.

Also, you might be a clinician or coach who is reading this, and I want you to have some more solid information than some stupid-ass blog about semen retention. When I talk about legal stuff later in the book, paraphilic disorders will be discussed again.

But, before that, some fun. In the next chapter, we'll get into some nerdy-sciency stuff about kinks and why we're into them. And we'll work on fighting back against both external and internal messages regarding sexual shame. Juuuuuuuust in case the gestapo is looking for a new book to burn.

Part One: Understanding Kink

WHY DO WE LIKE WHAT WE LIKE?

*I*t wouldn't be a Dr. Faith book if we didn't start by science-ing the fuck outta the topic. Also? Y'all are my fellow nerds who like that shit, and there might be a revolt if I skip that section. So let's talk about the brain science around getting turned on in general and getting turned on by kink more specifically.

The Brain Science of Horniness

It might not be the least bit surprising for you to learn that how sexual behavior is regulated by the brain is . . . really complicated. Sexual behavior is regulated by both cortical and subcortical structures of the brain. This means it's governed not just by the thinking brain but also by the feeling brain and the basic staying-alive functions of the brainstem and spinal cord.

And yes, the systems that produce dopamine and serotonin are definitely involved. But other neuropeptide transmitter systems, including the adrenergic system and the cholinergic system, are involved too. Essentially, our sexual selves are influenced by our whole-body systems, because sex is both primitive and complex. As well as both flexible and rigid (that's what she saiiiiiiiiiiiiiiiiid).

Now, how all of this fits together has been explained in many different ways. The one I'm going to cover in this chapter is the super well-known four-part sexual response cycle, which breaks down how all of these processes work together dynamically. Later on, in Chapter 3, I'm going to discuss another model, created by Rosemary Basson, which is helpful for figuring out what you like if you aren't exactly sure.

The Sexual Response Cycle

This model, which was developed by sex researchers Masters and Johnson back in the '60s, helps us better delineate the changes (both physical and emotional) that happen in our bodies when we are enthusiastically participating in sexual activity. Paying attention to our own bodies' responses can help us better connect with our partners and also figure out where/when/how things don't work as well as we'd hope (we'll be getting deeper into both of those topics in Chapter 3, so stay tuned). There are four phases:

Desire

Arousal

Orgasm

Resolution

Now everyone is different. Across genders and across humans. The timing of these phases and how long a person spends in each one differs from person to person and situation to situation. And you may not even go through these phases in this order, which we will look at more closely in Basson's model. For example, someone may seek connection and intimacy and may initiate sex with a partner for that reason, rather than starting with desire.

This doesn't make anyone bad or wrong or broken. This is just more information about how we connect to ourselves and others, based on what we notice during our experience of any of these phases.

Phase 1: Desire

Muscle tension increases.

Heart rate and breathing are elevated.

Skin becomes flushed.

Nipples harden, and individuals with more breast tissue may find that the tissue becomes fuller.

Blood flow to the genitalia increases, which results in swelling of the labia minora, vaginal walls, and clitoris if you have a vulva, and testical swelling and penile erection if you have a penis.

Lubricating liquid may begin to secrete, from both vaginae and penes.

Phase 2: Arousal

All changes that started during Phase 1 become more pronounced.

The vagina continues to swell and may even turn a darker color from the blood flow.

The clitoris becomes even more sensitive, to the point of being painful.

The testicals pull up into the scrotum.

Breathing, heart rate, and blood pressure continue to rise.

Muscle spasms in the extremities (face, hands, feet) may occur.

Muscle tension throughout the body increases.

Phase 3: Orgasm

Sadly, the funnest phase is also the shortest. This phase generally lasts only a few seconds, though longer for Sting, according to Sting in the '90s.

Blood pressure, heart rate, and breathing are really high, and you're needing to take in a lot of oxygen.

Involuntary muscle contractions begin, including in the muscles of the feet.

The muscles of the vagina contract, and often also the uterus.

Contractions at the base of the penis begin, which leads to ejaculation (the release of semen).

Sexual tension is released forcefully and suddenly (you know, an orgasm).

Flushed skin ("sex flush" or "sex rash") may appear over the entire body.

Phase 4: Resolution

This is the phase where the body returns to baseline.

All the body parts that have swollen and become more rigid return to previous size and color.

Heartbeat, breathing, and blood pressure return to baseline.

There is usually a sense of well-being, satisfaction, and also fatigue. Sometimes individuals feel emotional and may be tearful. Sometimes the physiological changes cause a headache or other secondary physiological response.

Some people are able to return to an earlier phase more quickly (these individuals are described as multiply orgasmic). Others need a longer waiting (refractory) period.

The Brain Science of Kinky Horniness

Ok, yeah yeah yeah. Now we know how the body responds to sexytimes in general terms, but why are some people hella vanilla, some people like to add a few sprinkles, and some people are comprised completely of sprinkles (and probably some assless leather chaps to hold all the sprinkles in).

First of all, let me say this: People being all weird, and different, and quirky, and bizarre makes me so entirely happy . . . shine on, my fellow weirdos, sexual or non-sexual. If you like to roll around in butter and call yourself a biscuit, that's fantastic, and you don't owe the world any defense of that behavior. It's fine, you're fine, and if you need me to pick you up some jelly when I run to the store let me know.

That being said, I'm going to go into the brain science around kink because it's so fucking interesting. And it can be an important part of destigmatizing kink in general and understanding your own responses.

How We Got Here: A History of Kink Research

But before we get into the current research, we need to do a little history lesson on how psychiatrists and sexologists understood kink, or "perversions," in the past.

The term *pervert* originally referred to a rejection of religious canon or religiosity. Meaning atheist. How did the term come to apply to sexual behaviors outside society norms? Three people.

First, there was Richard von Krafft-Ebing, the psychiatrist who is considered the father of our modern thinking on sexuality. At a time when sexual differences were criminalized, he was claiming that they were the product of mental disorders. Early in his career that applied not just to actions that were violent and non-consensual, but also to homosexuality. Again, he didn't believe these things should be criminalized; instead, he thought they should be addressed through psychoeducation on sexual deviancy and moral hygiene. And eventually he got over the notion that homosexuality belonged in this category. So we appreciate someone who can learn and grow.

But it also was super helpful when sexologist and scholar Havelock Ellis and literary critic John Addington Symonds wrote a book about homosexuality called *Sexual Inversion*, which was published in 1897. The book was accessible enough to general readers for the term *pervert* to enter the common lexicon. But Ellis and Symonds weren't being negative about homosexuality; they were pointing out the normalcy of queerness across species. Symonds actually came out as gay at a time when one didn't do such a thing.

Ellis and Symonds were also demonstrating that these "perversions" weren't actually problems, it was just that members of modern society considered them crimes against canon. Or, a rejection of a particular dogmatic religion. Ellis, while not a gay man, was equally open about his urophilia (yes, you guessed it, an adoration of golden showers). *Sexual Inversion* was a game changer that captured public attention at a great time. It was published two years after Oscar Wilde's famous indecency trial where he was sentenced to two years of hard labor for engaging in sodomy with Lord Alfred Douglas.

In the many years since Krafft-Ebing, Ellis, and Symonds paved the way for a shift in our thinking about sexuality, researchers have continued to demonstrate, over and over, that there are a helluva lot of kinky humans running around out there. In a study published in 2017, researchers in Quebec, Joyal and Carpentier, surveyed individuals specifically around the paraphilias listed in the DSM. It was a non-clinical random sample of people . . . meaning not people already in any kind of mental health services. A solid half of them reported interest in at least one of the paraphilia categories, and 30% had at least dabbled in one. And? They found evidence that this was a good thing. The people who were specifically interested in and engaged with masochism reported higher satisfaction in their sex lives.

And Covid didn't shut any of that down. In fact, a trend survey conducted by the dating app Bumble in 2022 found similar results. Almost half of the participants stated that they were approaching sex and intimacy with a willingness to explore. An openness to trying some different things from the menu, if you will. Of those surveyed, 20% said they had been actively doing so in the past year. And more than half of the respondents agreed that no matter what you are into, it's important to put all that on the table early in the relationship—that we should be open about our wants and needs and not waste our time with people who have fundamentally different ones. We'll get more into how to communicate about these wants and needs in Chapter 3, but for now, the big thing to remember is that being into weird stuff is pretty common and actually not weird at all.

Ok, Blind Me with the Science Then, Doc

So thanks to a long history of research on the subject, we now know that a lot of people are kinky. But what exactly causes this?

First of all, studying the etiology of anything is difficult. Because people continue to run around being people-y and subverting all expectations. And we can't do actual experiments to see if we can *create* a paraphilia in someone. Not any experiments that would be approved by an institutional review board, anyway.

So the bulk of research in the area is qualitative stuff. Like interviews, case studies, narratives, and questionnaires. And we are asking people not just about their behavior but their inner lives. And even the most open and honest people aren't going to get everything right. Plus, since so many people have guilt and shame experiences around their sexual appetites, we are likely not getting even the to-the-best-of-their-ability full story. That being said, we have picked up some great insights over the years. And while most of it is research like the above, once we start connecting these qualitative dots, some more experimental designs are also possible, like measuring blood flow to genitalia (and you thought *your* job was rough, right?).

One thing that researchers found pretty quickly was that when it comes to kinks and fetishes (outside of BDSM, which is the one area where all genders have a pretty equal interest in exploring), the sex-different ratio is huge: 99 out of 100 fetishists are (cis) men. The research on animals does show some sex differences that can help explain this. It demonstrates that some features of animals' development (not even traumatic ones, per se . . . just life experiences) imprint in a way that wires into their arousal patterns. Sexual imprinting, to be specific.

In humans, our best guess is that the age period that we think of as being fairly asexual is actually the time when male sexual imprinting occurs. And while we can shift behaviors, the imprinting itself appears irreversible. Some scientists believe that this is partially a function of the Zeigarnik effect.

The Zeigarnik effect is one of those little brain quirks that posits that we remember disrupted experiences more than experiences that we participated in to a satisfying completion. We remember not the Monopoly games that we played nicely until someone won but the games where someone yelled and flipped the board and accused the banker of cheating.

In terms of the development of more creative and interesting sexual behaviors, the idea is that the bright, inquisitive, and intuitive kids who are curious about and exploring sexual feelings are often silenced because we have an overall culture of shame around sexual expression that suggests this isn't an appropriate thought process for children to be engaging in. And the denial of their curiosity leads to imprinting on something that may not generally be considered sexually provocative.

Of the case studies we do have, there are several where the developed fetish was tied to something that was interesting to the individual during childhood. And in terms of brain science, what fires together wires together. I've shared the story before of a friend whose interest in rope play came from how much he loved Western novels when he was little. A lot of these novels had a scene where a woman was tied to the train tracks and had to be rescued from the bad guys by the good guys.

The stories were exciting and fun to read, and he would be breathless to get to the maiden's rescue. And all that intellectual curiosity and engagement in these stories is now part of his sexual operating system. He reports that his interest in rope play is about the aesthetics, not the power dynamics. Which makes sense based on his awareness of his childhood connection to these stories. As evolutionary psychologist Jesse Bering wrote in his book *Perv*:

> Like every other slot machine, this one has its own preprogrammed algorithm for randomizing the results. The only difference is that this algorithm involves a mix of factors that, together, will determine the individual's sexuality: genes, prenatal experiences, brain chemistry, early childhood events, family dynamics, cultural milieu, and an untold number of other inscrutably interacting variables.

Twin studies of paraphilic behaviors, where one twin expresses them and the other doesn't, also support this notion. Even with shared genetics and shared home environments, we still develop differently. Researchers point out that these individually meaningful confounds have a causal association with fetish behaviors. Which is how fancy science people say "things that happen to us sometimes cause fetishes."

It may seem disconcerting to consider that what we experience, traumatic or not, at an early age leads to an imprinting that cannot be eradicated. But while it may be an unwanted part of the human experience, it's actually a feature, not a bug. This level of imprinting enhanced men's chances of survival. And our understanding of this comes from the work of psychiatrist and researcher James Giannini. In 1998 he published his findings around podophilia (yes, the eroticisation of feet) as a sociosexual trend in relation to outbreaks of venereal diseases.

Sexualization of the female foot can be seen to have spiked during the gonorrhea epidemic in the 13th century, the syphilis epidemics of the 16th and 19th centuries, and the AIDS epidemic of the late 20th century. Shoe styles that showed more of the foot were popular, and feet were more prominent in art of the time, even. The interest would wane along with the outbreaks. Giannini posits that if men had an interest in a safer body part (syphilitic sores don't hide between toes), then they would have less contact with parts of the body that could carry an infection, which could lower their chances of illness and death—another likely mechanism of imprinting experiences.

And I know, I keep saying men. Why are women different? Cis women are known to show more *erotic plasticity*, both in qualitative studies and in studies that measure blood flow to erogenous zones. Erotic plasticity means that women can have a sexual excitement response to a wider range of stimuli. While men get locked into that specific target early in life, women's sexuality is far more fluid, even when we have specific likes and dislikes. Both straight and queer women (and again, these are studies of cis women) show vasocongestion (blood flow to the vagina, as we discussed in the section about the sexual response cycle) even in response to things they really aren't into.

We don't know if imprinting is due in part to more testosterone in the system[3] or if whatever imprinting we do experience is simply easier to override, but either way, this *also* makes evolutionary sense. Explaining this means I have to go a

---

3 This wouldn't be that hard to do some research on. If 99 out of 100 known fetishists are cis men, the 1 woman out of 100 could be tested for having more naturally occurring testosterone, which is common for a variety of reasons, including many intersex conditions. While the data would be correlative, not causal, it would lend some support to my pet theory. Someone with some NIH money should get on this.

little dark for a minute. Historically, in many cultures, sex was quite often an action that was done to women, not with women. We rarely had choices about sexual couplings. And Meredith Chivers's protection hypothesis posits that the physiology of the sexual response cycle (blood flow, fluid release) is designed to help prevent injury to our bodies. There will be less pain, tearing, bruising, and damage if we are able to physically respond with arousal (Phase 2), even if we find something intellectually or emotionally unappealing. Because, once again, this response is a feature, not a bug.

To this day, women report to me the shame and confusion they have felt when they've experienced arousal and even release during non-consensual sexual acts. Understanding why our physiology is at odds with our true desires is often instrumental to our healing. I think all of this research on the psychology and physiology of our sexuality is important, not just because it's hella interesting, but also because it's helpful for unraveling so many of the "thou shalt nots" related to sexual expression. We're just people being people-y. Our experiences of ourselves and our bodies are part of that being-human experience. And while some of our behaviors may be a problem if we aren't able to find healthy outlets, our attractions themselves shouldn't be.

UNFUCK YOUR SEXUAL SHAME

*B*ack to our beloved evolutionary psychologist Jesse Bering for a moment. He points out, pragmatically, that we are all perverts—that, trust, there is something you've either done or entertained that would engender a negative response in certain people if they knew about it. Which leads to an experience of shame. And over a century after *Sexual Inversions* was published, Dr. Bering (another out gay sexologist . . . I don't know if he is also a golden shower aficionado, we will have to ask him) is also endeavoring to look closely at the sexual shame experience and "smother it with reason" by pointing out that what is determined to be perverted is just us being human.

And when we spend so much time getting wrapped up in deciding what is "normal" sex and what are "perversions" . . . we are focusing our moral-panic energy on the wrong fucking things. Instead of focusing on sexual desires that are hurting no one, we should be focusing on things that should cause real moral outrage. Like racism, war, food scarcity, and impending social collapse.

This doesn't mean every behavior should be condoned. We're talking about understanding behaviors, not encouraging limitless and universal support for all of them. I used the phrase "hurting no one" early and I meant it. If you are into squishing your toes in butterscotch pudding while doggy-bobbing your partner(s) and everyone involved is into it, no harm is being perpetrated. Alfred Kinsey (yes, the superfamous sex researcher guy who also was kinky af) noted that "there is practically no other behavior which is forbidden on the ground that nature may be offended, and that nature must be protected from such offense. This is the unique aspect of our sex codes." This was a very polite way of saying that when it comes to sex especially, we have a tendency to decide that something is wrong without any evidence of it causing any harm.

Jonathan Haidt developed the term *moral dumbfounding* to explain the determination to maintain a specific judgment despite all lack of evidence. But it is also a little more than that. People believe stupid shit with no good reason in all kinds of arenas (hi, politics). But Haidt was specifically studying moral outrage and the circular logic of declarations such as "It's wrong because it's weird." In research studies where information is presented that shows that all avenues of all forms of measurable harm have been eradicated, study participants still default to a presumption of harm. We assume that a thing has to be harmful if we determine that thing to be wrong. Like Kinsey said, we view these things as crimes against nature itself.

So what can we do about these moral panics? How can we break out of this shame-based thinking about our own desires and behaviors? The first step is to become aware that this is what's going on. And then we can try to reframe our thinking. Many times I have asked clients who are in distress about their behaviors the following question:

If the world changed suddenly and no one cared about what you're into . . . would you still feel bad about it?

Meaning, say you like to masturbate while wearing finger puppets on each finger and listening to Wagner, and you're distressed about it because it seems a little weird. If you understood the world around you to be at least neutral on the topic of masturbating with finger puppets and Wagner, would you still be distressed by your desires? Or would you go forth with the thing you like?

Detangling Trauma Responses from Kink

Don't roll your eyes at me, you know I can't write a damn thing without talking about trauma. And seriously, oftentimes we think something we're into must be related to a trauma response, which then leads us to believe that we are doing something wrong and bad. And that we are fundamentally broken for doing it. Like if you have a history of experiencing abuse and you like BDSM, does that mean you're fucked up? And while the answer is generally no, it's super important to figure out why it's not a trauma reaction and what to do in the cases where it is.

First, the good news. The very good news that I want to say right off the bat (and that I will go into in more detail in the BDSM section of this book) is that there is *no* evidence that any kink practices are an unhealthy response to abuse or other incidents of trauma. In fact, when I went to check to see if that had changed any since I'd last combed through the research, I found *more* evidence that kink is *healing* to traumatic experiences and *still* no research indicating that it's reinforcing trauma responses. Which isn't to say it never happens. It's just far more rare than you'd expect.

In Chapter 5, I'm going to dance around with much excitement while telling you all about how healthy BDSM dynamics can be incredibly empowering and beneficial for individuals and their relationships. This is where most of the research lies, in part because BDSM is associated (incorrectly, but we'll get to that later) with violence and aggression, and in part because it's the one place where interest isn't divided by gender.

But while I'm a "let your freak flag fly" therapist, I am also aware that our expressions of sexuality can become entangled with our trauma history, and that is a really difficult thing to parse out. Of course kink can also be a problematic behavior, because anything can. And although there isn't much research around kink specifically, there is other research on trauma-propelled behaviors, which are generally referred to as *trauma reenactment*. The phrase trauma reenactment (along with the phrase repetition compulsion . . . another ungreat expression) is used to describe a pattern of recreating and repetitively reliving traumatic events from one's past. It's not a simple issue with a singular cause, because life is complicated and humans are complicated. Harvard (fancy!) psychiatrist and researcher Michael Levy has operationalized four main mechanisms of trauma reenactment. They are:

Mastery Posture: Meaning, we are compelled to reenact these experiences in order to better make sense of them and/or resolve them; this is a direct reenactment that reinforces the traumatic nature of the event. It is when we are stuck in an intrusive memory loop of the horrific thing that happened to us. In my practice, this is overwhelmingly common.

Adaptive Defensive Posture: This is where we reenact certain behaviors to gain better control over them and our responses, but we do so in a healthy way. Think of just about any superhero origin story, where the superhero in question went through a terrible experience as a young person and wants to protect others from the same. Batman and Spiderman both lost family members to violent crime and worked to protect others from that same loss, right? I

Maladaptive Defensive Posture: This is where we reenact certain behaviors to gain better control over them and our responses, but we do so in ways that hurt others . . . often in the same ways we were hurt. This is what's happening when the individual that was abused goes on to abuse others.

Rigid Defensive Posture: This one is really interesting because it isn't really about a symbolic engagement with our past traumas. Instead, it means our traumas have impacted us to the point that our sense of safety is based on maintaining tight control over how we interact with the world. A good example of this would be someone who struggles with avoidant attachment. If you are rigid in your determination to not be hurt by someone, you choose people to which you don't have to demonstrate any emotional availability. Researchers still consider it a reenactment of sorts, because it's an avoidance of any situation that we perceive as possibly harmful based on our trauma history.

So if anything, when we're talking about a relationship between trauma and kink, we are generally talking about an adaptive defensive posture. Meaning a healthy way of working through our ish. If we appreciate Batman, we can appreciate ourselves for making the best of things—for finding out life can be a pile of shit and looking for the pony, instead of just wallowing in it. If you're not sure? Here are some of the questions I use with individuals who are concerned that their trauma histories are being activated instead of healed in their sex lives:

1. Are the activities you are engaging in (doing, watching, thinking about) enjoyable in the moment or does it feel like a compulsory exercise?

2. After engaging in these activities, do you feel a sense of enjoyment/relaxation/pleasure or primarily a sense of relief?

3. Do these activities engender a feeling of playfulness/fun/connection or a sense of obligation?

4. When you are unable to engage in these activities due to lack of access or your own choice, do you feel like you are missing out or do you feel a sense of relief?

5. If you are not engaging in these activities, how do other aspects of your life fare? Do you feel more connection and enjoyment or less?

There is a bunch of complexity here, and this is likely an area where figuring this out on your own may be incredibly difficult if not impossible. There are so many brain systems and physiological responses in play that it's an incredibly tricky issue to navigate. Working with a clinician who is trauma-informed (not just vaguely trauma-aware) and has a level of training in human sexuality (rather than just being vaguely sex-positive) may be important. You may also need to experiment with behaviors to see what best supports your journey. What happens if you take a 30-day break from a specific type of porn, for example? What changes do you notice in your life overall? What about within your sexual expression? What have you lost and what have you gained?

Hypersexuality Doesn't Exist (At Least, It's Not Really a Problem If It Does)

The idea of hypersexuality is connected to all the other common ways that kink is treated like a shameful practice. Let's start with the frustrating news that there is continued advocacy for wanting hypersexuality to exist as a DSM diagnosis. In 2012, Harvard physician Martin Kafka led a group that advocated to have the DSM formally recognize hypersexuality.

First of all, let's be clear that he was really trying to create a diagnostic category around client distress and their subjective view of themselves. Which of course is important . . . it's *the* most important consideration. Additionally, his definition was based solely on the amount of sex someone was having, not the kind of sex. His definition was "excessive expressions of culturally tolerated heterosexual or homosexual behavior." Hookups, porn, masturbation, camming, chaturbating, that type of stuff.

His focus was on the distress the client was feeling about their behaviors, and their subjective negative view of themselves and their sex lives. This is admirable because it is a client-led paradigm, but the client's feelings don't exist in a vacuum. Our cultural values around what is appropriate are influencing our thoughts about our own behaviors, even if the only measure we are talking about right now is frequency. One of the influencing factors that has been the most studied is the impact of religious upbringing on sexual expression. Religious upbringing plays a moderating role in distress about "hypersexuality" . . . most people who seek treatment belong to an organized religious institution and report that their religion is important to them.

And please let me say, that isn't a problem in and of itself. I'm going to be deeply unthrilled with you if you tell me your religious upbringing prevents you from baking a cake for a gay wedding . . . but if you tell me you feel closer to your creator and happier and more content in your life if *you* don't engage in certain behaviors, then you have absolutely every right to abstain from them. I may be a huge fan of that particular behavior in my own life, but this ain't about me, right?

But a lot of people have some detangling to do around two competing identities that they are trying to make sense of, *which is a huge part of what we do in therapy*. It's not about forcing someone to leave their church *or* forcing them to stop having sex in a washtub of cream of mushroom soup. It's about figuring out their personal value system and how these other practices align or don't align with their best life.

Which is how we get to the APA disagreeing that this should be a disorder added to the DSM. Because it's just . . . figuring out life. And we need to not disorder every damn thing. Otherwise I'm going to need a hypericecreamality diagnosis and a manual of coping skills for not eating all the damn (dairy-free) ice cream I can get my grubby mitts on.

This isn't to say paying attention to the quantity and quality of sex people are having (and how they feel about it) isn't important. Human behavior exists in such a wide range, it's helpful to have some ideas around it. Which is how we figured out that churchgoing can be an issue if you are also butt-stuff-going and the like. But it is STILL just a number. And the number of engagements in consensual, non-harmful behaviors doesn't carry any moral weight. *Because no harm is being perpetrated.* Back to our evolutionary psychologist bestie, Jesse Bering, for a second:

> "One person's sexual exorbitant is another's slow Monday morning."

Dr. Bering also points out that the researcher's own idea of what's normal tends to influence the research around hypersexuality. As Alfred Kinsey once remarked, "A nymphomaniac is someone who has more sex than you do." So if the researcher in question thinks sex a couple of times a week is the "right" amount . . . someone who has 10 times that amount of sex would be concerning to them. And if the researcher considers their own desire range "normal," it means that someone having much more desire is "abnormal," which foundationally just isn't true.

The idea of hypersexuality has also led us to do horrific things to people for the sake of "curing" them. Did you know one of the original uses of radiotherapy was to burn away the clitoredes of teenage girls to prevent them from masturbating? We associate female genital mutilation with the continent of Africa, but we were doing the same thing in the US and England, because helping yourself to a solo orgasm implied you were deeply disturbed.

And this does also relate to kink. Even though the call to add hypersexuality to the DSM wasn't tethered to kink overtly (which, again, I appreciate) . . . it would end up getting tethered to kink functionally. Because research also shows that people with higher sexual appetites are the people who are more likely to engage in kink. Think about it like this: If you go to a great restaurant a couple of times a month you will likely order your favorite dish, or one of a couple of favorites. If you eat there far more regularly, you're far more likely to want to experiment with other items on the menu and less fearful of disappointment, knowing you can come back another day. It works the same way with sex.

Now if hypersexuality seems to kick in overnight? That is something to pay attention to. Hypersexuality as a flipped switch can be the result of a neurological condition, including the following:

Rabies

Tourettes

Multiple sclerosis

Huntington's disease

Klüver-Bucy syndrome

But again, that's only if you notice a sudden change. Most of the time, there's no pathology involved.

Sex Addiction and Porn Addiction Don't Exist

I have *many* people come to see me because their behavior regarding sex or porn is really pissing off their partner. The word "addiction" starts getting thrown around, and the doer gets an ultimatum that shit's over if they don't get therapy for their "problem."

Cheating, high sex drive, porn usage, masturbation, and other behaviors around sex have been increasingly attributed to sex addiction over recent decades. Sex addiction is a multibillion-dollar treatment industry . . . based on something that literally doesn't exist.

There is one thing that needs to be said first: Wanting sex, enjoying sex, and being excited about sex does not make you a sex addict. Having cheated on a partner means you did something shitty to someone you love, but it doesn't make you a sex addict. Wanting porn, enjoying porn, and being excited about porn does not make you a porn addict.

Let me say that one more time for the people in the back: *Being sex- and porn-positive does not an addiction make.*

A therapist shouldn't diagnose you with a sex or porn addiction, because the diagnosis doesn't exist. And according to the research, there is simply no such thing (if you are interested, check out my recommended readings at the end of this book).

The reason for this is that a so-called addictive behavior doesn't compute the same way when there is no physiological dependence and the consequences don't seem as severe. (As an aside, all those numbers being thrown around relating porn usage to divorces are entirely made up by anti-porn crusaders.) Sex- or porn-related behaviors *could* fall under the domain of "process addictions," which means there is no involvement of a substance that creates a literal physical dependency (like alcohol, nicotine, and other drugs), but the behavior itself has addictive qualities.

The problem is, when the brain lights up in the process of doing something like shoe shopping or gambling, it's easy to see the reward circuit being activated in a way it doesn't for someone who doesn't share that process addiction. But sex (solo or partnered) is SUPPOSED to light up the reward centers of the brain. EVERYONE'S brains light up that way. So can you safely label it an addiction? No.

Now, can someone engage in sexual behaviors that harm their relationships and other life domains? Sure. But it is very important to call it what it really is. *Dismissing problematic behaviors as addictions is a denial of responsibility and a declaration of a lack of self-control.* And that right there is some fucking bullshit. Anyone who is engaging in problematic behavior around sex is absolutely accountable for their behavior and absolutely able to recognize their urges and consider how acting on them will impact their partners and their lives in general in the long term.

So what can you do if you are worried that you may fall into the category of problematic sex or porn usage? There are a few good self-assessment tools you can find online. Use your Google-Fu to check them out. I've had people come to my office and announce a number they got from a self-assessment, and I've told them I don't give a shit. The point isn't to get a particular score that gives you a diagnosis, but to start a conversation. I use the answers to help them discover patterns of behavior in order to create better strategies around the actions that are causing harm.

Here are some more questions to consider:

Is sexual activity itself (either partnered sex or solo sex that is porn-stimulated) more important than your relationships—for example, your relationship with the person with whom you are having sex?

Does it take the place of true connection?

Are you experiencing a lot of life stress right now? Or depression or grief or anything else that's really difficult to deal with? And have you started using sex or porn more than usual as a coping skill?

Are you skipping out on other important things in your life because of your behavior around sex or porn? Be honest . . . were you late to Grandma's birthday dinner because you were all engrossed in Xtube last weekend?

Are you feeling out of control of your behavior, instead of seeing sex or porn as another way of expressing who you are as a person? Like, is it costing you money you don't have or causing legal consequences?

Is sex or porn something you use for connection and/or fun, or is it a compulsion you fight with every day?

Is your behavior at odds with what your partner thinks is appropriate? Your church? Your family? Your community? Is this about other people's core values or your own?

Here is the big thing I want you to look at: how sex and porn either hinder or support your relationships. In the end, all addictions are replacement relationships. (And while problematic use of sex or porn isn't actually an addiction, this feature still applies.) They become more important than the people that we love. They become more important than ourselves and prevent us from being human beings out there connecting in the world.

Problematic use of sex, masturbation, and/or porn comes about when the thing we are doing becomes more important than all of our reasons for being, and our behaviors are drained of meaning and context. Obviously, people who are unhappy with their usage of sex and/or porn don't like what they are doing. Not past the immediate moment of engagement, anyway. And they don't like themselves all too much either. Because their behavior is separating them from all the amazing, messy, authentic, beautiful relationships the world has to offer, it's no longer aligned with their values, and it keeps them from prioritizing the people they love. That's what defines a problem.

If you realize that your current sexual activities are posing a problem for you, then you may benefit from getting some support. One of the biggest problems in this area is the number of clinicians who have ended up profiting on the stigma and shame surrounding sex. Which means that doing careful research will be really important. Ask any therapists that you are interested in seeing what their stance on sex addiction and porn usage is. If you are dealing with past religious or cultural messages around your sex and pornography usage, ask them if they are comfortable helping you explore that without adding their own value system to the conversation. I recently read an article by a therapist who views masturbation as a form of spousal abuse. Yes, literally. People are out there spewing that kind of nonsense, and there is enough shame and stigma around sex as it is . . . you sure as fuck don't need it from your therapist.

Look, Let's Talk about Porn in a Little More Depth for a Second

The internet has been incredibly helpful for increasing access to and consumption of porn. While the internet was developed for the military-industrial complex, it quickly privatized for porn (Rule 34 of the internet shows up yet again, sorry Al Gore!). Through a process that sex researcher Alvin Cooper referred to as the triple-A engine effect, it offers affordability, access, and anonymity. According to 2010 statistics, 40 million Americans are regular consumers of porn. And a solid third of those individuals are women. Of all the websites in existence at any given time? 12% exist for porn.

Ok, but before we start yelling about parental controls and how the sky is falling and the like? We should note that while we have more porn access, the number of wank-a-thons hasn't changed. In the '40s, Kinsey started tracking the total sexual outlet of men (TSO, I kid you not . . . which means, yes, shot spooge . . . through either partnered or solo sex) and the Kinsey Institute has continued to track these numbers. The number of times a man has an orgasm, on average, has remained stable. Even with more relaxed attitudes and increased access to porn, we have about the same amount of sex and wanks as we did in the '40s. Additionally, even back then the amount of sex we were having was seen as problematic. Kinsey found that according to prevailing standards, 75% of men were hypersexual.

But hey, are we fucking up our kids with all this porn exposure? Current research does show that the average age of first porn exposure in Western society is about 11. So first of all, I am pre-internet old. I saw my first pornographic materials when I was younger than 11. *Playboy* magazines abounded. We all knew whose dad kept them in the house and where to find them. We all saw them for sale at garage sales. We all knew that one older kid who had a couple pilfered away in a treehouse or fort. I remember thinking, "Huh, ok, adults are kinda weird." I definitely wasn't traumatized by it.

The difference between my youth and that of my kids is that while I grew up in a sex-positive, education-forward household, discussions about the normalcy of porn and masturbation were nascent. It was treated not as a bad thing but as a joke thing. My kids were raised knowing that it was normal, healthy, and natural. That it might even help your cranky mood and definitely could help take the edge off if you had a date with someone you were really into and you wanted to not get too excited and pushy. Discussions around porn in my household (sorry, my now-grown kiddos . . . you're getting invoked again) included explaining that it was a form of art like anything else, designed to be viewed and enjoyed, and therefore wouldn't be as similar to sex with a partner as you might think/hope/fear. And that erotic performance work is WORK, and should be paid for just like anyone else's work. So if anything, my kids grew up with a healthier understanding of porn than I did.[4]

As for the complaint that the internet has bred new kinks? Let's go back to Rule 34 of the internet ("If it exists there is internet porn of it"). Nearly all paraphilias predate the internet, and it is far more likely that the internet served as a means to pull marginalized people together and help them find their community. Whether it be fellow queer kids who grew up in evangelical churches, or fellow people who like to wank into red ski caps. Rule 34 of the internet is really just Rule 34 of life, because humans are kinda slutty.

What about all those (poorly designed) research studies that demonstrate that porn is causing erectile variability? Better-designed research studies found that an increase in performance frustrations was related not to pornography viewing . . . but to the common human experience of anxiety. A stressed-out nervous system is not going to be great at upregulating our physiology in the ways necessary to experience the completion we were hoping for (read: have an orgasm). Remember all the stuff that happens throughout the stages of sexual excitement? There's a lot going on that can be influenced or subverted, and when we expand our

---

4 Don't worry, I messed them up in other ways, I'm sure.

research to look at other aspects of someone's life, we figure out that porn is really not the problem.

So here is where sexologists and sex therapists get rowdy and start organizing like the orcas. There are all these pornography abstinence programs out there, sold (at very expensive prices) by these anti-porn groups. And their existence is stupid. But people spend money on stupid shit all the damn time, so why do we care about these useless programs? Because when participants fail (and they generally will), failure invokes suicidality. Because the meta-message associated with these programs is that you are bad and wrong for self-lovin', which has biological importance beyond just feeling good.[5]

And porn usage has demonstrated really interesting positive results, which I am geeking out over sharing with you. I don't just mean qualitatively, like people saying, "Look, I dig it and it's not a problem." There's also more concrete evidence that the anti-porn crusaders are just fucking wrong. Here's how we know. From 1948 to 1989, the Czech Republic was under a communist regime and there was a total ban on porn of any kind. Not just "pure" porn but also erotic books and magazines, etc. If it was vaguely smutty at all, it was a no-no.

When the communist regime fell in 1989, the country entered its villain era. Which meant wilding out quite a bit. And? Complete deregulation and decriminalization of all kinds of porn. And biologist Milton Diamond thought, "This is a scientific experiment just happening in front of us . . . sweet," and tracked

5 Especially all y'all humans with a penis. Another important feature-not-bug of the human body is that it ensures that we have fresh ejaculate available. Because the point of ejaculate is baby-making. And old semen is more likely to lead to birth defects and the like. So the body gets rid of it regularly. So if you aren't having partnered or solo sex, you're going to end up having nighttime emissions.

what happened. Other crimes went up because people had been under decades of police-state action and they had partying to do. But the rates of sexual abuse against children and sexual crimes against women dropped *enormously*.

The access to these different types of porn allowed viewers who had proclivities in those directions to experience them without hurting anyone. The porn was cathartic. This has also been found to be true in Japan and Denmark. Individuals who have desires that would cause harm if acted out report that having this access gives them the release they need so they don't harm a human being.

So it's not just that people enjoy viewing sexytime media for their own sexytiming, and that it can help with stress, anxiety, and all those other human frustrations. It's also that porn prevents crime—horrifying crimes against the people who need the most protection. Yes, you can find studies about the harms of pornography. But look at who is sponsoring the study. Look at the study design. Did the researchers pay attention to the ways the porn was a positive or neutral influence, or did they just focus on harm? The practical suggestion made by many sexological researchers is to continue having porn available for all taste levels. Especially when technology, AI and otherwise, allows us to create porn without human actors that could be harmed in the process (see Chapter 6 for more on ethical porn consumption).

Advocate for Real Harm Prevention

When we are talking about the things that may cause harm, understanding and compassion can help us better prevent that harm. The question isn't whether a sexual desire or behavior is natural or unnatural. The question should be "is it harmful to anyone involved?" And if there is no harm, all these moral panickers need to take several fucking seats or spend their excess energy volunteering at a soup kitchen.

And having a specific interest, even to the point of having a diagnosable paraphilic disorder, doesn't mean you offend. Most people that have sexual interests that would intrude on another individual's sovereignty are horrified by these desires and work very hard to never hurt anyone. Meaning they know that what turns them on would be an offense against someone else. So they do not commit that offense. They seek out fantasy play, porn, and other outlets in order to meet their sexual desires in a healthy way.

But this can be difficult for people to understand, because humans hate wrestling with complexity. We want complicated problems to have simple solutions and they just fucking don't. So if banning drag shows won't do anything to lessen sex crimes, that means we have to wrestle with complexity despite how exhausting it is to do so.

We need to inculcate real harm-prevention skills with our littlest humans (you know . . . teaching this shit in school, like they do in many other places in the world), and we need to approach therapy and coaching and other mental health spaces with lots of psychoeducation around dealing with our own processes and finding safe ways to meet our sexual desires. And we could start by addressing the actual issues we know are associated with sexual harm.

So what are the commonalities among people with paraphilias who do offend? A study focused on individuals in the US and

Canada found four, so let's go into what these characteristics are and how we can address them to prevent harm.

High moral disengagement: Moral disengagement is a term developed by Albert Bandura to describe the inner justifications we come up with to explain away our shit behavior. This is when we claim that there are extenuating circumstances that allow us to act in terrible ways. Interestingly, research shows that we may do this not just before we make a decision but also afterwards, in order to avoid the heavy lifting of accountability work. Working with this behavior means encouraging reflexivity and accountability. It means fostering a culture that embraces and encourages change work by inviting in rather than calling out, and that embraces grace instead of blanket cancellation toward the people who are doing the work.

Impulsivity: Any clinicians that study approaches to out-of-control sexual behaviors outside the addiction framework will tell you screening for neurodivergence is one of the first things we do. This is because undiagnosed or unmanaged ADHD is strongly associated with problematic sexual behaviors, since the executive function skills needed to manage our impulses burn out pretty quickly. So we have to screen for (and, you know, TREAT) those underlying issues.

Higher sexual excitation moderated by lower sexual inhibition: Addressing this means giving individuals with higher sex drives means of release that don't cause harm, as well as helping them learn skills to inhibit the harmful behaviors.

Maladaptive understandings of consent: You know when I will stop including materials on consent in everything I write and teach? When I no longer have to. Cuz damn, this is a big one. I feel like I am fighting the tides of shitty modern media that (still!) bulldozes consent in order to maintain a cute storyline. I know plenty of really lovely, thoughtful people who have histories of not taking consent seriously because they were literally taught otherwise. You know what I mean, right? The people who were told they had to be a little bit pushy, because playing hard to get is part of the game. It isn't (nor should it be) a game. So how do we counter this? It starts with better education on what consent is and isn't. See Chapter 4 for a longer discussion on this topic.

I'm including all this information because y'all are my people. You are equally exhausted of simplistic ideas and bullshit solutions. You want fun things to stay fun and everyone to be safe and respected. And this is our starting point in advocating and teaching and raising awareness in our own communities, because what we need is more education and thoughtfulness on these subjects, not more shame.

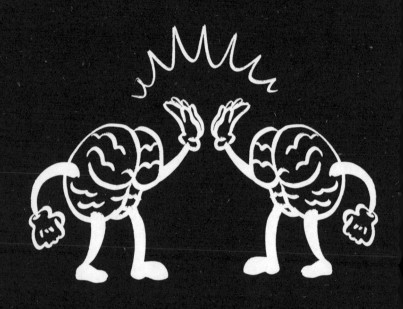

COMMUNICATING ABOUT WHAT TURNS YOU ON

S o a big takeaway from the last couple chapters is that every body operates differently and there is no one right way to experience sexual pleasure.

Ok, I take that back, there is. The one right way to experience sexual pleasure is to communicate clearly with your partner (if partnered sex is your thing) and then enjoy the agreed-upon plan together.

And there is no way to talk about it without just talking about it. Just like the only way out of Mordor is through Mordor. It can be uncomfortable, whether y'all are brand new or been together a minute. Though as uncomfortable as it feels, it becomes far easier and more natural with a little time. Because with very few exceptions, your partner is going to know their body way better than you do. And the resounding theme of the rest of this chapter is "here is an idea . . . if you and your partner are into it."

So other than admitting you were reading this book (which could be a great start), how else can you open up the conversation? A lot of my couple clients (and throuple and so on, FWIW) have found that using a yes/no/maybe checklist (which helps you sort out what you're into, what you're not into, and what you're unsure about) is a solid way of opening up the conversation. But before we even get into that, a lot of peeps also really benefit from starting with an identity conversation. Not just the standard "my name is [blank] and my pronouns are [blank]," but getting even more specific about how that relates to their body and their sexual expression. While this is hugely important with someone new, it also may be helpful to re-open this dialogue and explore these questions with someone you have been with for some time. Because sexuality is so fluid, they may have new things to share with you, or you with them. This format is one I modified from a yes/no/maybe checklist written by Tab Kimpton as part of the Khaos Komix series.

Identity Information

I describe my gender as:

My pronouns are:

My gender descriptor words (e.g., femme, butch, boi) are:

My sexual-orientation identity words (e.g., lesbian, bi, queer) are:

My sexual role words (e.g., top, bottom) are:

My terms for my chest or breasts are:

My terms for my genitals are:

My terms for my prostate or Gräfenberg spot are:

My terms for my anal region or alimentary canal are:

Pick one: These terms are relatively static for me **OR** These terms are relatively fluid for me.

If they are fluid, this is how I communicate that information to a partner so they know to shift language:

Some words I am not ok with to refer to me, my identity, or my body, or that I am uncomfortable using or hearing, are:

I am activated (and not in a good way) by the following words or language:

Are certain words ok in some settings or situations but not in others?

How so? (Explanation optional; you can just include which situations your partners should watch for.)

How flexible am I with my preferred terminology? What if my partner wants to use a different term for something?

Any other important information to share?

Yes/No/Maybe Checklists

Great! Next helpful part? Sharing with a partner or partners what you're into. Checklists can be helpful tools for this. These checklists can be super intricate, involved, and intensive, and many of my clients have reported back, "Ok, so I'm not kinky at all, considering all the possibilities out there." So trying to create an inclusive one here is pretty impossible. Also, there are really good checklists already available, including ones that are more specific to different interests and one that is specially designed for visual communicators. The last one on the list is specific to consensual non-monogamy. Check them out online and see if any feel like a good starting place for you:

Sexual Interests Checklist (AskingForWhatYouWant.com)

Yes/No/Maybe List (SexWithEmily.com)

Yes, No, Maybe So: A Sexual Inventory Stocklist (Scarleteen. com)

The Super Powered Yes/No/Maybe List: A Negotiation Tool for Sex Nerds (BexTalksSex.com)

Navigating Consent & Setting Sexual Boundaries: Yes/ No/Maybe List (SunnyMegatron.com)

You Need Help: Here Is a Worksheet to Help You Talk to Partners about Sex (Autostraddle.com)

Poly Yes/No/Maybe List (Polynotes.tumblr.com)

But What If I Don't Know Enough about Myself to Know What Turns Me On?

As frustrating as it feels to be in a situation where you don't know what gets your engines revved, please know that you are far from alone and you are miles away from unusual. We think of sexual desire as something that someone gives us. That is, it's someone's job to turn us on.

That's an oversimplification of how contextual desire really is.

In reality, our sexual expression comes from something within us that we, in turn, can choose to share with a partner. Rosemary Basson's sexual desire model[6] demonstrates that before we get to actual sexual desire, there are several steps in the process that are about our internal world and our connection to our erotic selves.

---

6 Dr. Basson's model is an explanation of the sexual excitement cycle of cis women. And while there are absolutely differences among the genders and just within humans in general, I've found that mindset and self-knowledge are important to everyone.

This model is helpful for all folx who experience themselves as more sexually reactive. It is really normal to not really get turned on until you're put in a sexy situation. Then you react to it with your own sexual interest. Most people don't go all hubba-hubba when just at the grocery store or whatever. I have worked with many people who think that they are somehow broken or dealing with unhealed trauma because their desires tend to be more reactive, and looking at the normalcy of that excitement pattern can be both helpful and healing.

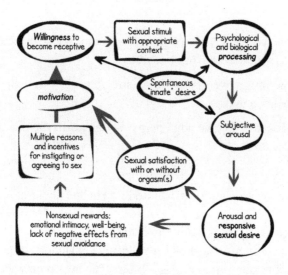

While expanding our repertoire and experimenting with new things is a fun part of being a sexual being, so is slowing down and connecting back to ourselves and what we like and don't like. It's another form of mindfulness. It means being curious within ourselves instead of judgmental, and letting go of the rules and assumptions we have created for ourselves and our sexual encounters.

This is all connected to the fact that consent is a continuous process that requires us to listen to our own bodies just as continuously (don't worry, we'll cover consent in more detail in the next chapter). What was right for you in the past, and what may be right for you in the future, may not serve you in the present.

Let's look at some questions to help you connect to that space:

When did you feel like your most authentic self (connected and grounded in your body)?

What things were you doing for yourself that helped facilitate that?

What activities give you energy or feel worth the energy they take?

What activities feel playful to you?

What gets you curious and interested in life?

Engagement through the Five Senses

Another way we can build a solid understanding of how we connect to our inner eroticism is by reflecting on how we most strongly engage in the world. We all explore the world through our five senses (or at least as many of these senses as we have access to), and we all tend to be more strongly engaged through one or two of them than the others. In her book *Urban Tantra: Sacred Sex for the Twenty-First Century*, Barbara Carrellas points out that recognizing which sense we most connect to can help us receive with more intentionality. So let's look at where you stand, yeah?

Visual
When you recall details about an event, do you most easily go to what you saw? How easily can you visualize your childhood home? Where you live now? What your favorite person looks like? Is how someone looks or how they move their body sensual to you?

Kinesthetic
When you recall details about an event, do you most easily remember how things felt when you engaged them with your body? How easily can you remember what your favorite article of clothing feels like on your skin? How it feels to pick up a warm mug when your hands are cold? The sensation of jumping into a pool of water? What a partner's body feels like when it connects with yours?

Auditory
When you recall details about an event, do you most easily remember what you heard other people say or noises that were made? How easily can you remember someone's tone of voice? How easily do you learn and retain information when it is told to you verbally? Do you most connect with the sounds a partner makes during sex?

Olfactory
When you recall details about an event, do you most easily remember what things smelled like? How easily can you remember what your elementary school classroom smelled like?

Your favorite flower? Your favorite perfume or cologne? Do you most connect to a partner's scent?

Gustatory
When you recall details about an event, do you most easily remember what things tasted like? Can you easily recall the taste and texture of your favorite food? Can you see or hear about something and imagine what it would taste like immediately? Do you most connect with how your partner tastes when you kiss or lick them?

If you are noticing some clear differences in how quickly and clearly certain memories come up based on one or two of your senses, this can provide some great cues on how you connect to your own sexual desire and how you share that with a partner. Practice engaging the world with these senses on a daily basis and with a partner, and see what new things you start to figure out about yourself!

After-Action Report
Any time you're engaging sexually with someone, and especially if you are being game to new experiences, unpacking the experience after the sexual response cycle is over can be incredibly beneficial. Is this something you continue to want on the menu or nah?

Do you feel relaxed? Happy? Calm? Embodied? Satisfied? If this is a person that you have a relationship with, do you feel closer to them? These are all signals of a positive experience.

Positivity aside, not everything has to add up to 100% amazing. It's also important to ask yourself what you enjoyed specifically: What brought you the most pleasure? What was less pleasurable? What was the most physically intense? Emotionally intense? Did anything surprise you? How so? Was there anything that you struggled to convey in the moment that your partner would benefit from hearing? Is there anything you wanted to share feedback on?

If you are struggling with some guilt afterward, check in with yourself about whose voice speaks this guilt. If it's external, question that. If whoever speaks with such judgment in your head was silenced (a family member, a pastor, society in general), how would you feel? If no one on the planet cared that you liked having sex while wearing an Eeyore onesie, and in fact everyone was highly encouraging . . . would you still feel that it was wrong? This helps us separate out cultural programming from our own authentic desire.

But . . . with trauma histories it can be difficult to figure out what is authentic to us, versus what is a ghost of past pain. If this is your history, check in with the specifics around that. Did you feel connected or dissociated? Was your entire focus on your partner or did you stop to connect to your own pleasure (because yes, giving is also supposed to be pleasurable)? If you find that you perform well with a partner but struggle with being truly present, I'd strongly, strongly suggest a therapist who works specifically with trauma, because you deserve authentic pleasure too!

Changes in Sexual Performance and Desire

I haven't met anyone who has a partner or wants a partner who doesn't also worry about sexual performance. Among those of us who engage in partnered sex, our sexual enjoyment is generally not selfish, but something we want to share with someone else.

We don't want our partners to think they are doing something wrong when our bodies aren't responding the way we would like them to. In reality though, human bodies can functionally derail pretty easily, and it has nothing to do with our partners. And since this sort of thing can affect anyone, no matter how kinky or vanilla they are, it's always helpful to understand what's going on with our bodies as part of figuring out and communicating our desires. So let's go over some of the physical factors that can change or interfere with desire and performance.

Sexual Dysfunction: More Than Just ED

Erectile dysfunction tends to get a lot of attention (we've all seen the Viagra commercials), and we'll talk about it in a minute. But people with penes aren't the only ones affected by sexual dysfunction, and there's a lot more to this conversation than just ED.

The term *sexual dysfunction* is an umbrella term used to refer to any problem anywhere in the sexual response cycle (motivation/desire, arousal, orgasm, resolution) that impedes our pleasure. Focusing for the moment on people with vaginas, issues that fall in this category include:

Anorgasmia: Inability to have an orgasm

Dyspareunia: Experiencing pain during sex

Hypoactive sexual desire disorder: Lack of desire, also known as low libido

Sexual arousal disorder: Problems with arousal

Research demonstrates that about 30–40% of individuals with vaginas and vulvas are affected by one or more of these issues, with low desire levels being most common. But as history has consistently shown regarding medical understanding of our bodies, there are likely some accuracy problems with these numbers.

Most of the arousal research has focused on genital congestion (blood rushing to the area and erectile tissue becoming erect) and lubrication, because those have typically been good measures for individuals with penes. But for those of us with vaginas, sexual excitement more often starts with thoughts and emotions. It's far more subjective than just a measure of vasocongestion.

Additionally, we are less likely to experience spontaneous desire and spontaneous sexual fantasies, and are more likely to experience our sexual selves as a part of ourselves we connect to, draw forth, and share with a partner (Esther Perel's book *Mating in Captivity* speaks to this further).

Low Libido

Let's talk a bit more about low libido. Libido exists on a spectrum. Not just among different people but even within ourselves. Low libido (aka hypoactive sexual desire disorder, impaired sexual function, diminished sex drive, etc.) is an issue with the mind-willing part of sexual expression. It's about the wanting to have sex, versus the physical excitement around sex (like an erection or lack thereof). The Mayo Clinic notes these signs of low libido:

Loss of interest in any form of sexual activity, both partnered and solo

Lack of sexual fantasies or thoughts

Feeling unhappy or worried about either or both of the above

This is a well-thought-out list of indicators because it really focuses on a change that is not perceived as positive. This allows for a distinction between people who have a desire disorder and people who are simply asexual, greysexual, or demisexual. But if you have low libido and you're miserable about it? It could be the result of many different things. Stress, drug and alcohol usage, not sleeping for shit, other physical and mental health conditions (hormonal changes being a big one), toxin exposure, relationship stressors . . . One of the other big culprits for both ED and low libido are medications, both over-the-counter and prescription. Medications that may cause these conditions are listed in the sections below, because that's the easiest cause to address. Speaking to your doctor about changing up your medications may resolve the issue quickly.

But it's important to remember that all medications operate in the body differently. They take varying amounts of time to take effect and to clear out. So not taking a medication or other substance for one day may or may not be an efficacious litmus test. Read up on whatever you're taking and talk to your prescriber about anything that they have given you. What are options for titrating your dosage or stopping altogether? Can this be done safely? What other side effects might occur that you need to watch for? When would you notice a difference? All that complicated adult-y stuff.

Medications That Can Lead to Low Libido
PRESCRIPTION MEDICATIONS:

Anti-anxiety medications based on benzodiazepines (Xanax)

Anticonvulsant medications (such as Tegretol, Phenytoin, Phenobarbital)

Antidepressants (including anti-mania medications, antipsychotics, MAOIs, SSRIs, SNRIs, tricyclic antidepressants)

Benign prostatic hyperplasia treatments (such as Flomax, Propecia, Proscar)

Cancer treatments (including radiation and chemotherapy)

Heart and blood pressure medications (including ACE inhibitors, a-Adrenergic blockers, b-adrenergic (beta) blockers, centrally acting agents, diuretics, thiazides, and statins)

Hormonal contraceptives (such as Ortho Tri-Cyclen)

Opioid pain relievers (such as Vicodin, Oxycontin, and Percocet)

Steroid medications (including anabolic steroids and corticosteroids)

OVER-THE-COUNTER MEDICATIONS:

Antifungals, specifically ketoconazole or fluconazole

Antihistamines, including Benadryl (diphenhydramine) and Chlor-Trimeton (chlorpheniramine)

Tagamet (cimetidine)

RECREATIONAL DRUGS:

This category is harder to listicle, because people's experiences with recreational drugs vary widely. Alcohol and THC are examples of super-common substances that elevate libido in some people and crash it out in others. So anything you are taking may be having a frustrating impact on your sex life.

Other Health Issues That Can Harsh Our Mellow:

Hormonal changes (thyroid hormone and prolactin are two big ones, as are hormones used for bodybuilding and the ones used to treat prostate cancer; we'll talk about hormone therapy in a minute)

Medical conditions (UTIs, etc.)

Vascular issues (anything that affects blood flow, particularly to the penis)

Other health conditions (diabetes, heart disease, high blood pressure, multiple sclerosis, arthritis, and anything that affects pain and mobility)

Depression (depression is a total libido killer . . . 50% of the individuals that struggle with major depressive disorder have sex drive, sex arousal, and even vaginal lubrication issues), stress levels (cortisol decreases sex drive), drug/alcohol addiction, trauma history (especially related to physical sexual abuse)

Toxin exposure (ugh, the inflammation)

Sleep disorders

A sedentary lifestyle (bodies really need to move, and if that isn't part of our regular daily activities, they get grumpy)

Body image issues and self-consciousness

Relationship problems in general

Erectile Dysfunction

First of all, erectile dysfunction (the experience of not being able to get or maintain an erection firm enough for penetrative sexual activity) is super common. Like, so common I really wish we would stop calling it a dysfunction and start calling it "another perfectly normal, albeit frustrating, thing that human bodies do." Sexologists often use the term *erectile disappointment*, which is more pithy and closer to reality than the word dysfunction. But we could use an explainer that is even more pithy and clever than that, so feel free to talk amongst yourselves and get back to me.

How ED is defined and then measured has so much variability, the numbers you will see will also vary wildly. (One study said that worldwide, between 3% and 76.5% of people with penes will experience it at some point in their life. Which feels like the scientific version of throwing spaghetti at the wall and seeing what sticks.)

Generally, though, the prevailing notion is that ED affects one-third to one-half of cis men at some point in their lives. And while it is associated with increased age and diseases like diabetes, I am seeing plenty of surveys showing that really young people are frustrated with ED. Like under-30 young. If this is you, you are by no means alone.

Just like with low libido, there are a lot of things that can contribute to ED, and medications are one cause that can be relatively simple to address.

Medications That Can Contribute to ED

ANTIDEPRESSANTS AND OTHER PSYCHIATRIC MEDICINES:

Amitriptyline (Elavil)

Amoxapine (Asendin)

Buspirone (BuSpar)

Chlordiazepoxide (Librium)

Chlorpromazine (Thorazine)

Clomipramine (Anafranil)

Clorazepate (Tranxene)

Desipramine (Norpramin)

Diazepam (Valium)

Doxepin (Sinequan)

Fluoxetine (Prozac)

Fluphenazine (Prolixin)

Imipramine (Tofranil)

Isocarboxazid (Marplan)

Lorazepam (Ativan)

Meprobamate (Equanil)

Mesoridazine (Serentil)

Nortriptyline (Pamelor)

Oxazepam (Serax)

Phenelzine (Nardil)

Phenytoin (Dilantin)

Sertraline (Zoloft)

Thioridazine (Mellaril)

Thiothixene (Navane)

Tranylcypromine (Parnate)

Trifluoperazine (Stelazine)

ANTIHISTAMINE MEDICINES (CERTAIN CLASSES OF ANTIHISTAMINES ARE ALSO USED TO TREAT HEARTBURN):

Cimetidine (Tagamet)

Dimenhydrinate (Dramamine)

Diphenhydramine (Benadryl)

Hydroxyzine (Vistaril)

Meclizine (Antivert)

Nizatidine (Axid)

Promethazine (Phenergan)

Ranitidine (Zantac)

HIGH BLOOD PRESSURE MEDICINES AND DIURETICS (WATER PILLS):

Atenolol (Tenormin)

Bethanidine

Bumetanide (Bumex)

Captopril (Capoten)

Chlorothiazide (Diuril)

Chlorthalidone (Hygroton)

Clonidine (Catapres)

Enalapril (Vasotec)

Furosemide (Lasix)

Guanabenz (Wytensin)

Guanethidine (Ismelin)

Guanfacine (Tenex)

Haloperidol (Haldol)

Hydralazine (Apresoline)

Hydrochlorothiazide (Esidrix)

Labetalol (Normodyne)

Methyldopa (Aldomet)

Metoprolol (Lopressor)

Nifedipine (Adalat, Procardia)

Phenoxybenzamine (Dibenzyline)

Phentolamine (Regitine)

Prazosin (Minipress)

Propranolol (Inderal)

Reserpine (Serpasil)

Spironolactone (Aldactone)

Triamterene (Maxzide)

Verapamil (Calan)

Thiazides are the most common cause of erectile dysfunction among the high blood pressure medicines. The next most common cause is beta blockers. Alpha blockers tend to be less likely to cause this problem.

PARKINSON'S DISEASE MEDICINES:

Benztropine (Cogentin)

Biperiden (Akineton)

Bromocriptine (Parlodel)

Levodopa (Sinemet, Carbidopa)

Procyclidine (Kemadrin)

Trihexyphenidyl (Artane)

CHEMOTHERAPY AND HORMONAL MEDICINES:

Antiandrogens (Casodex, Flutamide, Nilutamide)

Busulfan (Myleran)

Cyclophosphamide (Cytoxan)

Ketoconazole

LHRH agonists (Lupron, Zoladex)

LHRH antagonists (Firmagon)

OPIATE ANALGESICS (PAINKILLERS):

Codeine

Fentanyl (Innovar)

Hydromorphone (Dilaudid)

Meperidine (Demerol)

Methadone

Morphine

Oxycodone (Oxycontin, Percodan)

OTHER MEDICINES:

Aminocaproic acid (Amicar)

Atropine

Clofibrate (Atromid-S)

Cyclobenzaprine (Flexeril)

Cyproterone

Digoxin (Lanoxin)

Disopyramide (Norpace)

Dutasteride (Avodart)

Estrogen

Finasteride (Propecia, Proscar)

Furazolidone (Furoxone)

H2 blockers (Tagamet, Zantac, Pepcid)

Indomethacin (Indocin)

Lipid-lowering agents

Licorice

Metoclopramide (Reglan)

NSAIDs (Ibuprofen, etc.)

Orphenadrine (Norflex)

Prochlorperazine (Compazine)

Pseudoephedrine (Sudafed)

Sumatriptan (Imitrex)

Recreational drugs:

Alcohol

Amphetamines

Barbiturates

Cocaine

Marijuana

Heroin

Nicotine

Age-Related Changes

Oh, my bouncing baby Buddha, save us from the idea that our sexual primes are in our 20s. And praise be to sex therapist David Schnarch, author of the book *Passionate Marriage*, for challenging the notion by pointing out that there's a big difference between one's genital prime and one's sexual prime.

Sure, our genital primes (the physicality of how our bodies function) are when we are younger. But our sexual primes? Not until way later. A study of men in Norway found that those in their 50s experienced more sexual satisfaction than they did in their 30s, even if not everything was as hard, wet, or quick to bounce back, or whatever else we may miss from our youth.

As we get older and have had more sex, we leave behind our exploratory years and enter the years of self-confidence. We know what we like. We know how we like it. We are exhausted of the insecurities that the larger culture has foisted upon us, and we have started living to be comfortable in our bodies. Which leads to better sexual encounters and orgasms. And if you feel that you aren't there yet? You're literally doing the research to help you get there, which makes you a total badass.

And yes, older generations are still having lots of sex. Even generations that came of age pre–sexual revolution. Because bodies do age and like to do wonky, non-behaving things sometimes, oral sex can become an even more integral part of sexual connection with a partner (read: penetrative intercourse can become more difficult to accomplish for a multitude of reasons). In studies of sexual behavior, older couples are more likely than younger couples to connect oral sex with improved relationship quality and overall happiness.

Physical Disabilities

Disabilities can be something we are born with (genetic) or something that happens to us later on (acquired). In both cases, there may be fuckery to overcome beyond living in a body that isn't performing the way you want it to. The cultural messages around disability (and the presumption that you now exist in the category of non-sexual) are slowly changing, though we still have a long way to go.

I think it's most important to note that while individuals with physical disabilities (especially those who struggle with day-to-day tasks without assistance or support) report engaging in mutual sexual activity less frequently than able-bodied folks, there are many factors besides frequency that predict sexual satisfaction and sexual esteem. One can have lots of sex and find it generally unpleasant and unfulfilling, right?

Additionally, the longer we live with the physical limitations of our bodies, the more positive we feel about ourselves as sexual beings. Just like we feel more comfortable with our sexual selves as we get older, we also have the capacity to grow into a level of comfort with our bodies over time.

Hormone Therapy

Despite what a neoconservative politician would have you believe, most of the people on hormone therapy are not doing so as part of gender-affirming care. Meaning most people on hormones are cisgender. For some people, hormone therapy can be a game changer in terms of desire, arousal, and performance. But because the brain is the biggest sex organ in the human body, our self-concept also has a huge impact on our sexual desire. Hormones change our entire bodies, and someone being on hormones for a thyroid condition, for example, may not feel great about how that changes their physical appearance, which can in turn affect arousal.

Additionally? If someone who is on the trans spectrum is on a hormone therapy regimen as part of their care, they may also notice changes in their arousal patterns and in how they perceive their body, which impacts sexual desire just as much as it can for a cis person.

Even if you are loving all of the health benefits of hormone therapy, you may find that your erogenous zones have changed, which is important to communicate about with a partner.

Part Two:
Exploring Your
Pervy Desires

AUNTIE FAITH SAYS, "MAKE SAFE(R) CHOICES! BE A RESPONSIBLE SLUT!"

Know Where to Get Your Information

*I*t's almost like some weird thing always happens to illustrate a point I'm trying to make. This time it was the "Bambi sleep files." Have you heard of the Bambi sleep files? They are a series of erotic hypnosis tapes made by an (as of this writing) anonymous individual designed to inculcate a personality that's super feminine, sex-obsessed, unsmart, and very obedient. The instructions in the tapes also demand the user forget the content of the listening sessions. And the tapes are awful. The "forget what you've heard" part is the antithesis of hypnosis ethics, and the tapes emphasize it over and over in their endeavor to turn women into flesh-and-blood sex dolls. There are statements like "a docile, unconscious dolly who accepts and forgets everything and any ability to counteract her deep bimbo programming."

Excuse me while I go shower the grossness off of me.

Ok, back. Dammit. Yes, there have already been reports of significant mental health problems associated with the use of these tapes. They are creating dissociative responses in individuals, which lead to consent situations that aren't truly consensual. There is nothing wrong with playing with one's own expression of femininity. Bimbofication as a form of role-play is definitely common in kink communities, and there is nothing wrong with that either. But it is not play if one is altered to the point that the consent is being forced, not given.

And I offer all this not just to warn you away from these tapes, but also to show that we need to be proactive around kink education and who provides it. We now have a trillion ways of connecting to the kink community through social media. And while connections are great, we are finding tons of misinformation that can be concerning or even downright dangerous. While normalizing and talking about kink is fantastic, learning physical skills really works better in a physical class. A video demonstrating binding someone's wrists with a belt is maybe not as dangerous as the Bambi sleep files, but learning these skills from a video leaves a lot of room for error and creates a high potential for injury (and here is me saying please don't do that).

If you are looking to explore something like this, I promise you will gain so much from going to an educational meetup, class, or conference. You can find stuff in your area by checking listings on FetLife (the largest, as of this writing, social network for kinksters) and asking at your local sex toy stores, sex clubs, and the like. Pay attention to whose names come up over and over again as good, safe, ethical educators. And if anything ever feels off or shady, dip on out of there. You're no Bambi except exactly when you want to be.

Embrace Consent

I've been writing and teaching on consent for far longer than it has been a buzzword in the ether. Now I'm going to blast you with it all over again in case you're new to the crew or could use a refresher because I am annoyingly persistent like that. Also? Further along in this book, when talking about legal issues with kink, I'm going to review a protocol that was specifically designed to prevent legal problems, using language that goes further than even our most thoughtful traditional kink models. So (insert evil villain laugh) even if you skip this particular section, it's going to come up again.

What Is Consent and Why Do We Need to Discuss It?

Consent is *the informed, voluntary permission given or agreement reached for an activity/exchange between two or more sentient beings.* Consent is generally how we communicate boundaries. If someone asks you, "Hey, can I borrow this book?" they are recognizing that the book is something you own (property boundary!) and asking if they can use your book and return it (consent for exchange!).

But consent is also an active process of communication. It's not just the *"can I [blank] this part of your body with [blank] part of my body"* that we see repeated ad nauseam in mainstream media. It's just as much my cat flattening her ears when she doesn't want pickie-uppies. Or my husband scrunching his face when I even *think* about putting onions in whatever I'm cooking.

At its core, consent is simply *permission for something to happen.* Consent defines our rules of engagement, the ones we express through boundaries.

We have all had experiences where our boundaries were violated and others did not request permission to interact with us, especially in regard to sex and intimacy. I am continually surprised/not surprised by how often even my fellow clinicians in the field misunderstand the need for active consent in relationships. People incorrectly presume that permission for one activity implies permission for others.

And a lot of us are out here trying to correct these misunderstandings, because consent is the key to providing a safe framework for interactions. For those of us with trauma histories, a safe framework can be a very healing experience. And, equally important, it allows us to experience our desires in a sex-positive way. In an ideal situation, you aren't having to be convinced, you're saying *yes*!

A Modern History of Consent

The concept of affirmative consent is often attributed to the authors of a policy put in place at Antioch College in 1991. It was a response to two occurrences of rape on the campus that year and a need for a more inclusive sexual misconduct policy. The policy spelled out that during sexual activity, everyone involved must give verbal consent to each activity that was being considered. Oral sex wasn't consent for anal sex, and sex on Tuesday was not consent for sex on Friday. It was met with great derision from the media . . . including an *SNL* skit that made fun of it (still findable on YouTube if you aren't old enough to remember it).

But actually, the idea of affirmative consent predates the Antioch College policy by a few years . . . and it comes from the kink community.

As HIV gained more awareness, BDSM communities started writing rules on *asking permission*. In 1981, the first formal bylaws regarding affirmative consent were written by members of a New York leather collective known as the Gay Male S/M Collective (GMSMC). They coined the term *safe, sane, and consensual*, a concept that is still used within the kink community (for an explanation of this and other consent-related terms that have been embraced by kink communities, check out the terminology section later in this chapter). Their work has been continued through the National Coalition for Sexual Freedom's Consent Counts Program. The Consent Counts Program currently defines consent as follows:

> For our purposes, consent is the explicit indication, by written or oral statement, by one person that [they are] willing to have something done to [them] by one or more other persons, or to perform some sort of act at the request or order of one or more other persons. In terms of sexual consent, consent may be withdrawn at any point, regardless of what has been previously negotiated orally or in writing.

The work of the kink community and Antioch College are the underpinnings of the letter the Obama administration sent out to 7,000 college campuses in 2011, challenging how sexual assaults were investigated by universities under Title IX. This letter, coupled with the Clery Act, a consumer protection act regarding campus safety and crime policies, started a shift in how we view consent and respond to violations of consent. In 2017, the state of California implemented a law requiring high school students to receive information on consent.

I've included this brief history of consent to give you an idea of where we've been and where we're headed. Thankfully, we've made some progress in how we understand and teach consent in recent years, but we still have a ways to go. The following sections will get into the nitty-gritty of what consent looks like, in kinky encounters and beyond.

The Consent Commandments

These 10 commandments came from a class I was teaching a few years ago for clinicians working with teens. We walked through group activities they could use to teach consent and boundaries *and* work with issues related to boundary violations. When it comes down to the basics, however, there are some fundamentals that apply universally. And as a good preacher's kid, I dug the idea of some basic commandments. Just like the OG commandments that Moses lugged down on stone tablets, they operate as a guide for our relational interactions, without weighing near as much, thankfully.

1. Consent for sex (and any other behaviors you are asking someone to engage in) cannot be given by people who are drunk. Or under the influence of drugs. Or hardcore medications. People under the influence are already doing seriously dumb stuff, like craving those two-for-a-dollar tacos from Jack in the Box. So don't add something to their regret list that has large, long-term consequences.

2. Going through a lot of emotional stuff can be just as bad for your decision-making process as being drunk. If someone is stressed out or dealing with a lot, they may be seeking comfort and connection, and we often equate

that with sex. If you think someone isn't making a good decision, put sex on hold and be there for them in other ways—like ones that won't embarrass them a week from now.

3. Consent isn't static. Agreeing to something on one occasion does not mean agreeing to it forever. So I let you borrow my car last week. Maybe you brought it back with the gas tank empty and full of used Starbucks cups and candy wrappers and I don't want you using it again. Maybe you took fantastic care of it, but I still don't want you using it again. Either way, it's still my car, not yours. You don't just march into my house, grab the keys off the counter, and take off in my car because I let you do it last week. A lack of consent equals grand theft auto, right?

4. Consent for one thing isn't consent for another. Someone gets naked in front of you? This is an excellent sign, yes. Is it consent for any specific sexual activity? No. Agreeing to one kind of activity isn't agreeing to all of them. Making out doesn't mean oral sex is cool. And yes to oral sex doesn't mean yes to penetrative sex. Our interactions are a salad bar, not a casserole. Wanting croutons doesn't mean you also have to have bell peppers, yanno?

5. Silence isn't consent. Someone may not actively say no, but being passive isn't a yes. Many times individuals don't speak up because they are freaked out or don't know how to. They could be quietly unhappy or quietly enjoying themselves. You don't know if you don't ask.

6. Consent needs to be informed. Are you sleeping with other people? That's ok—it's called dating, not getting married, for a reason. Have a sexually transmitted infection? That happens, too. Moving out of state in a week? That can impact future plans a bit. Potential partners need to know all of the above and any other information that may inform their decision about sexual activity. Be grown-up enough to have the awkward conversations.

7. Consent is a community obligation, not just a personal one. We need to help support each other with gray areas of consent. Speak up if you see someone in an uncomfortable situation and back up their right to say no. Friends don't let friends listen to Nickelback, and they don't let them get into situations where they are not really giving consent or not really getting consent. If you see someone at a party getting into a danger zone, then be the protective wingperson. And if the DJ plays Nickelback, it's time to leave altogether.

8. Having to convince someone is not consent. You aren't trying to win a court case by wooing a jury member. You're awesome, right? If they aren't into you enough to realize that and you have to convince them, then they don't deserve your awesomeness. If you get a "Welllllllll, I don't knowwwwww," respond with, "That's cool, let me know if you change your mind" and then step away from the sex.

9. Consent doesn't just mean the right to say no; it also means the right to say *yes*. Shaming people because they choose to engage in sexual activity makes active,

enthusiastic consent way more complicated. Affirmative consent is difficult for many people (usually women) because they think that an enthusiastic yes means they are slutty, and that they are supposed to pretend they *don't* want sex and must be "convinced." This sends mixed messages to their partners. When are we supposed to "convince" and when are we supposed to just stop? If everyone is sexually empowered, no one ever has to be "convinced."

10. Consent is about more than just sex, it's about boundaries in general. You should get people's permission to touch them for any reason (e.g., "You look like you could use a hug right now, would you like one?"). Consent extends past physical boundaries, as well. You should never force your will on others. Don't share others' information, experiences, images, or things without their permission. Don't make plans on their behalf without their permission. Don't force them to share information with you or anyone else if they are uncomfortable doing so. No matter what you think is in their best interest, unless you are their legal guardian, let them make their own decisions. You do you and let them be them.

Types of Consent

We've started having more conversations around sexual consent in recent years (yaaay!), but they have been pretty stuck in a thematic loop of "active continuous consent or nothing!!!" when in reality it's far more complicated than that. Having real discussions around consent means understanding our cultural norms (and dismantling the fuck out of them as needed). So let's dig into those.

Originating consent is a philosophy term that refers to our cultural standards of acceptable behaviors. It's the societal understanding of what is a legitimate and appropriate practice and what is not. Originating consent is fluid, as cultural context is ever-changing. What that means is that our laws come into effect based on our cultural standards of being good humans to each other.

Shifts are made when people start saying "What the fuck is up with this?" and laws are put into place to back that up. Laws, ethical standards, and the like are almost always *historical*. Meaning, we create them when we realize there is a problem that needs to be addressed. In England, it became against the law in 1275 to "ravish" a maiden (with or without her consent) if she was not of marriageable age (which was 12). That's when social norms of originating consent were formalized into laws. The law against raping children was formalized once people realized that raping children was a problem that couldn't be ignored.

Far more recent example: the term *upskirting* refers to the practice of taking photos or videos of someone literally up their skirt without their consent. In 2016, a grocery store clerk named Brandon Lee Gary went to trial for doing exactly this to a woman who was shopping at the store he worked at. His conviction was overturned in appeals because the law didn't reflect the illegality of this boundary violation (technology allows for creativity in shitty behavior). Courts don't make the laws, they only interpret and uphold them . . . so the next year, the Georgia legislature passed a bill into law that made upskirting illegal.

Originating consent is an important part of any boundary conversation because that's where cultural shifts are recognized and formalized into law as need be. You've heard the term *consent culture*, right? Consent culture is the normalization of asking for consent for interaction with others. Of being disappointed but not butthurt when someone says no. Consent culture at its highest level is when we don't feel weird or embarrassed for establishing and respecting boundaries. Our shift to consent culture means we are shifting our understanding of originating consent. And as our thinking shifts, our laws are starting to reflect these ideals.

About motherfucking time.

Ok, so now that we've all earned an advanced degree in philosophy, let's talk about what originating consent looks like in regular life.

Permissive consent is another term from those wild kids in the philosophy department. Permissive consent is what allows us to engage in specific actions in relation to those cultural standards of practice and social norms. For example, originating consent holds that it is not acceptable behavior to stab needles into another human being on the regular, right? But if you go see a tattoo artist, sign their waiver, and pay them for their work, you are engaging in *permissive consent*.

Permissive consent is our expression of boundaries in context. And despite all our conversations about active, continuous consent, the reality is that most consent is *not* verbal. This isn't good or bad, it's just something to be aware of.

Permissive consent is established in one of three ways:

- **Explicit consent** requires the yes to be spoken or written. It is directly expressed consent. A contract that is reviewed, understood, and signed before an exchange is explicit consent. Asking another person "may I _____ your _____" is explicit consent. When we talk about active, continuous consent (meaning active agreement to activity with continued check-ins to make sure the activity is still a go), we are talking about explicit consent.

- **Implicit consent** operates on presumptions of nos and yeses. It is the inference of consent based on our actions and circumstances. This isn't a fundamentally terrible thing. We do it all the time. If I purchase a bag of pistachios and leave it on my husband's desk, the implication is that they are there for him to eat. If you apply for a job and your resume includes the names and contact information for references, the implication is that the potential employer will call them to verify your employment eligibility. This is also the area that gets people in the most trouble, such as when someone presumes that engaging in one sexual activity implies consent for another activity that wasn't discussed.

- **Blanket, opt-out, or meta consent** are types of consent that require a no to be spoken. They give the opportunity for the no, and if the no is not forthcoming, the yes is presumed. This is another common way of operating within close relationships. For example, someone you know well may hug you when they see you, and the presumption would be that that is a norm in your relationship. If you weren't down for a hug, you would say "I'm super touched out today, I need a rain check on the hug" to let them know there needed to be a change in your normal interactions. An example within the BDSM community would be in edge play (see Chapter 5 for more on this), where the dom is setting the scene but the sub has a safe word that they can invoke. Consensual non-consent (pretending to say no when y'all already decided it was part of the play) would also likely fit in this category. Another common feature of BDSM scenes is role-play that mimics forced activity. Meaning pretending to not consent during the scene when consent was agreed upon beforehand. For example, maybe you're really into the idea of your partner being so turned on by you that they just come in, rip off your clothes and take you straight to poundtown. If y'all agree to role-play that very scene, with you yelling "No! Wait!" or other things that would mean "stop your shit right fucking now" in regular circumstances? But it's an agreed-upon part of the role-play before it starts, and there's a way for each person to stop the scene if they need to? Then you're practicing opt-out consent. Makes sense, right?

Some Consent Terminology

Just like the concept of affirmative consent in general, these terms were born within kink communities but are hugely beneficial in all kinds of situations and interactions.

- **Age of consent** is a legal term that varies by country and by state or region. It refers to the legal age an individual must be before they can legally engage in and consent to sexual activity. In some countries (like Bolivia), the age of consent corresponds with puberty. In others the age is in older adolescence, such as in the United States, where it lies between ages 16 and 18, depending on the state. There are sometimes exceptions to age-of-consent laws, such as within marriages that were performed with parental consent.

- **Capacity to consent** refers to an individual's ability to understand the activities they wish to engage in, as well as to make and communicate decisions about those activities. Someone may say yes to an activity but may not have the capacity to take responsibility for that yes if they are under the influence, or if they have certain developmental limitations or mental health issues.

- **Informed consent** refers to the consent that is given freely and willingly by another party once they have been given all pertinent information about what they are agreeing to, before the action takes place, without any pressure, coercion, or misrepresentation of the situation. You must also be of the age of consent and have the capacity to consent in order to give informed consent.

. . . and some BDSM-specific consent terms . . .

- **Good, giving, and game (GGG)** is a term that was coined by Dan Savage, a US writer with an internationally syndicated sex column. This term describes individuals who have no problem expressing their sexuality and are willing to try new things, within reason and with the expectation that boundaries are respected. GGG folks have worked through previous negative messages about sex and embrace sexual pleasure as a rightful part of their lives. Outside of sexual interactions, being a GGG person means embracing all the unique qualities that make you who you are, not being ashamed of your quirks, not being interested in toeing the party line, and finding the people with whom you can connect authentically. GGG people are not ashamed of geeking out over the current season of *Dr. Who* or a new recording of Wagner's *Der Ring des Nibelungen*. You do you.

- **Safe, sane, and consensual (SSC)** is another term from an alternative-sexuality community referring to the components required for consent. SSC was adopted by the BDSM community to differentiate between BDSM and abuse. Safe means that all risks involved in the interaction are understood by all parties and everything possible is done to reduce or eliminate those risks. Sane means that everything is done in a realistic way, and everyone can effectively differentiate between fantasy and reality. And consensual remains the basis of all interaction—it means that all participants were in an appropriate frame of mind to explicitly consent to the activities being engaged in. SSC easily applies to all relationships, not just sexual ones, because the fundamental message is to be mindful and thoughtful in our interactions with people.

- **Risk-aware consensual kink (RACK)** evolved as a response to the term *SSC* in order to recognize that some BDSM activities are not always risk-free. We'll go deeper into this one (and its potential legal complications) in the next chapter.

- **Personal responsibility, informed, consensual kink (PRICK)** became a more common term around 2009, according to the website Kinkly, as part of a response to concerns around the acronym RACK. This is another one we'll discuss more in the next chapter.

Consent in Conclusion

I know. That was a lot. Talking about consent is always a lot. But it's so important, and I hope this section of the book helps you be more mindful and purposeful in your interactions with others as you continue on your kinky journey. Remember all the research about what separates out offenders and non-offenders? And how not understanding consent was a big predictor that someone would offend? And how I threatened you with the foreknowledge that I was going to go over consent once again just for that reason? This was that reminder. Most of us aren't used to having and expressing agency in our lives, so practicing autonomy and choice in intentional ways can help us create huge shifts in how we interact with others while respecting them and ourselves.

STI Prevention and Safety

You might've thought we were done discussing all the safety stuff and ready to move on to the fun parts, but I'm not finished going all sex-educator auntie on you. I am from the generation that went into adulthood only to find out that sex—even vanilla sex—could kill you. While that is far less likely to happen nowadays, at least in the Western world thanks to antiretrovirals, Auntie Faith would still prefer for you to not have to manage the complexity of an STI, no matter what kinky stuff you're into. So let's take a moment to talk about all the protective measures.

Firstly, if you are not in a closed relationship where everyone has been given the all-clear, please please please glove your love. And consider both pre-exposure prophylaxis (PrEP) to way reduce your risk of getting HIV and post-exposure prophylaxis (PEP) if you aren't taking PrEP and you have a barrier-method failure during sexytimes.

And here's a note on oral sex specifically: Whether you're using barrier protection or not, don't brush your teeth for two hours before or two hours after oral sex. While your attention to oral hygiene is deeply appreciated, keep to a nice mouthwash gargle, because brushing does create bleeding gums and microabrasions in most of us, and that becomes an entry point for all kinds of cooties. Even if blood is part of your kink, let's keep the germs out.

Now, as for barrier methods? There is plenty of stuff on the market, no matter what kind of sex you're having.

Along with condoms (both internal and external, and let's not forget the flavored variety), we have gloves and finger cots (which can be specifically helpful for oral sex after metoidioplasty, as well as for fingering) and sex dams, which are placed over the vulva or anus during oral sex. Additionally, a Malaysian gynecologist recently released a condom created from adhesive surgical dressing that can be used in a multitude of ways (innies, outies, and all-aroundies). One hack that Auntie is cool with? While condoms cannot be DIY'd, sex dams can! A condom can be cut open to create a dam (and while you don't want to use a spermicidal condom for oral sex, you can use one for a dam conversion, so long as the spermicidal part isn't where your mouth is going).

Dental dam
(used on vagina and anus)

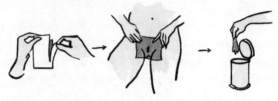

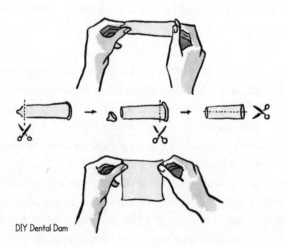

DIY Dental Dam

Disposable gloves (which make manual sex safer on its own) can also be converted into a dam by cutting off the fingers and then cutting open the palm of the glove along one side and unfolding it. But even easier? Barrier dams made from plastic wrap have proven to be effective in preventing the spread of STIs. Super easy.

Another trick for sex dams that I picked up from the *Scarleteen* website is to write a non-reversible letter, number, or symbol on one side of the dam so you don't accidentally reverse the dam later during play. You could even get creative with this and write something that ties into a kinky scene you're doing.

And don't forget to also take safety precautions when using sex toys as part of your kinky adventures (yes, that includes using barrier methods with toys). But there's a whole section about sex toys in Chapter 6, so I'll save those details until then.

Be Hella Aware of Legal Issues

While society is slowly limping along in recognizing that kink behaviors, especially BDSM, are not inherently harmful, that recognition hasn't made its way to the legal system yet, where these behaviors often continue to be pathologized. A recent case involved a man who had been convicted of strangling his live-in partner and then handcuffing her to their bed. She passed out from the strangulation, at least briefly, which was something that had also been agreed upon beforehand. It was done as part of a BDSM scene that was consensual on both their sides, but the court disagreed in 2020, and the Oregon Court of Appeals upheld part of the conviction in 2022. Within the original trial, the judge told the jury that in cases of strangulation, "consent or non-consent is simply not a factor," thereby essentially ensuring the man's conviction of strangulation and assault.

The appeals court judge did overturn the assault conviction but let the strangulation conviction stand, stating that the state legislature only allows for three contexts in which strangulation is not a crime: medicine, dentistry, and religious practices. Now, I have definitely known some shitty doctors, dentists, and clergy. None of them strangled me, and I'm not sure under which conditions them doing so would be acceptable, but ok??? Regardless, since the law doesn't have any language that states any flexibility around strangling-just-cuz-you're-into-it, the ruling essentially codified BDSM as an illegal activity.

This isn't the first or only case where BDSM itself was put on trial, just the most recent. It's also not just a US thing, even though we do often suck in our own unique ways. In the UK, a three-year investigation called Operation Spanner, which began in 1987, resulted in the prosecution and conviction of gay men engaging in BDSM behaviors while being filmed.

At first the police thought it was a precursor to a snuff film and started an investigation. The participants in the video got wind of this and reached out to the police to explain it was a BDSM scene, everyone was still alive, and no one participating needed any kind of medical care for being involved. It was BDSM being BDSM, sorry to scare you, Mr. Officer! Mr. Officer did not agree and pressed charges against 16 of the participants for "assault occasioning actual bodily harm." Which, since you read the earlier part of the paragraph, we know *did not happen*.

Again, the courts ruled that the consent of all parties involved was "immaterial" in a "civilized society."[7] The convictions ranged

---

7 Also? I'm fucking sorry, but if you are so civilized, let's start with the British Museum returning all the Indigenous artifacts that were looted by colonizers, shipped back to Europe, and put behind glass for others to look at. Pretty sure civilized societies also don't support theft?

from fines to prison sentences and were upheld through appeal after appeal, including in the Court of Appeal, the House of Lords, and the European Court of Human Rights. One of the judges in the House of Lords stated:

> I am not prepared to invent a defence of consent for sadomasochistic encounters which breed and glorify cruelty.

While the BDSM community has been thoughtful and considered in providing safety practices for decades, these guidelines haven't filtered into the areas of legal protection. We've talked a lot about consent among the individuals involved, but we also have to understand that we may not be able to prevent legal system intervention as long as those in power continue to consider kink a crime against nature itself. So let's go over some potential legal complications of a kinky lifestyle and what you can do to avoid them.

Even FOSTA-SESTA May Enter the Chat

In 2018, a pair of laws known together as FOSTA-SESTA (Fight Online Sex Trafficking Act and Stop Enabling Sex Traffickers Act) went into effect. They came from a place of wanting to protect victims of trafficking but instead put many other individuals at great risk.

Including me, y'all.

After the legislation passed, I went to a class provided by a lawyer for all of us who work with human sexuality. It was a mixed group of sex workers and body workers, as well as coaches and therapists like myself who only *talk* about such shenanigans. The lawyer's warning, which proved to be prescient, was that the new legislation did little to help real victims and instead put all of us at risk for being in or near the orbit of human sexuality. The broadening of definitions around sex work and a changed definition of trafficking means that even my private practice website could be tagged as sexual content, therefore opening me up to legal ramifications.

The immediate effects on sex workers were chilling, and a topic for a different day. The parts I want you to be aware of are that if you work with professionals as part of your kink engagement (like paying someone to dominate you or quite literally *anything* where money changes hands), there is a new level of legal risk involved. Also? The broadening of the definition of the word *trafficking* includes *any paying off of someone's debt*. So if you loan some money to your professional dom, say, with the plan that they will pay it off over time either in cash or in services? You just trafficked them, according to FOSTA-SESTA. And as is almost always true when we try to tighten laws in response to moral panics, the actual sleaze—real traffickers and coyotes—continue to cockroach their way to continued survival.

Possible Legal Issues around Paraphilic Diagnoses

So the DSM was intended to be a shorthand tool to facilitate communication between treatment team members. If you have a diagnosis of bipolar disorder, for example, anyone else you work with will have an understanding of what that means in terms of your symptoms and support needs. However, the DSM has also long been used by the court system to make legal determinations about someone's continued connection with the justice system. Meaning, how much the courts are going to fuck with them. This is especially true in reference to the paraphilic disorders, which have been used to engender extended (and sometimes even lifelong) psychiatric commitments.

The problem is this: the courts generally differentiate between non-pathological sexual violence and sexual violence that is the result of a paraphilic disorder, meaning there's an ongoing mental abnormality that creates a concern that there will be additional victims. The reworded definition of pedophilia in the DSM-IV resulted in two unanticipated problems related to this. Several groups (most of which were conservative and religious) were unhappy with the DSM-IV criteria, stating that it meant that pedophilia couldn't be diagnosed as a mental disorder unless it caused the individual in question a level of distress. That was a valid point, so the DSM-IV-TR (TR stands for "text revision," meaning this was an updated version) reinstated the wording of the DSM-III-TR for all the paraphilias that involve non-consenting victims (pedophilia, voyeurism, exhibitionism, frotteurism, and sexual sadism [why sadism was included, since it doesn't correlate to non-consent, I don't know]).

So now we had the phrase "or behaviors" back in the DSM criteria. Which led some forensic evaluators to conclude that any sexual offenders qualify as having a mental disorder based solely on the fact that they committed an offense. So let's say . . . you're drunk at a street fair and can't get to the porta-potties, so you pee in a bush. Public indecency charge unlocked, right? So you complete your public service or your 30 days or whatever the judge smites you with. Then? In more than 20 states, you could be civilly committed to a mental hospital after you serve your other sentencing requirements because you have been evaluated as having a "mental abnormality" that makes you a continued danger to society.

The authors of that section of the DSM-IV-TR published a piece a bit later saying, essentially, that that was absolutely not their intent and they understood that not all sexual offenses are related to a paraphilia (in fact, most aren't), and this wording issue should be fixed in the DSM-5. So fast-forward to today? It hasn't been. Nor is it corrected in the DSM-5-TR. A good forensic evaluator will be well-versed in these changes and will spend considerable time accessing other sources of information about patterns of behaviors and other possible reasons for the individual's actions.

Which is all to say, this is another area where being a non-shitty weirdo may get you tagged as a shitty one, with epic consequences. Whether you catch a case, or you have some diagnosis on record and you are currently going through a divorce and custody arrangement or *anything* that involves the legal system? There could be horrifically far-reaching consequences. Be proactive and nosy about any assessments or evaluations or therapy you undergo, and pay attention to how you are diagnosed. And my clinicians? Please be hella careful about assigning one of these diagnoses . . . you may be not just shorthanding a treatment approach, but creating a lifelong problem for someone who is just a run-of-the-mill kinkster and is of no danger to the larger community. And also please, please, please check out my resources list for some support for your evaluations.

Lessening the Chance of Catching a Case

Please know that the chances of this happening are pretty fucking rare. But I would be remiss as a sex educator if I didn't mention that it is possible, and there are things you can do to lessen the risk even more.

While we talked earlier in this chapter about consent for sexytimes in a more general way, I am going to run back around to this again, because if you are getting into a kink territory where the law may not be understanding (hell, many states don't even have a legal definition of consent on the books), going a bit further in your consent strategies may afford some protection against prosecution. Within the kink community, this extra-crispy version of consent+, developed through a partnership between the National Coalition for Sexual Freedom (an organization I have been a member of for years . . . and if you work in the field of human sexuality, you should be, too) and the American Law Institute, is known as *Explicit Prior Permission (EPP)*. EPP requires explicit informed consent, a kibosh on extreme behaviors, and the ability to end activities at any point in the process. Their model uses the language of both criminal and penal codes, as it was designed specifically for the types of behaviors that may garner attention from the justice system. EPP has five components:

1. Everyone participating is in agreement about both the acts you are going to engage in and the intensity of them. With *specificity*. "I'm going to cuff you and have my way with you if you're down for that" doesn't cut it for an EPP agreement.

2. You are of sound mind. Meaning you have the capability to consent. If you are a minor, you can't consent. If you are altered for any reason (meds, drugs, alcohol, heat sickness . . . whatever), you can't consent. If you are legally considered a vulnerable adult? The court system may discount your consent.

3. You can't seriously injure someone. Piercing play and some other types of activities have to be monitored so

fucking carefully because the chances of injury aren't minimal.

4. Everyone involved has to understand what resistance is part of the play and what is true resistance. As in plan ahead of time. Is saying "No, no, please stop!" part of the game while "Ow! Fuck! I'm out!" is not? Safe words and safe signals should be reviewed here.

5. Everyone involved has to be able to stop the action at any time. Remember the case from Oregon where the man strangled his partner and she passed out? Once she passed out, she could no longer stop the activity, right? Even if she had said ahead of time that yes, it is fine to ravage her unconscious body, that is a big legal no-no. You have to be capable of consent and you have to stay capable of consent during the whole scene.

The authors of EPP also strongly suggest that consent be given in writing (not just through verbal and nonverbal communication) and that it be updated for each scene . . . even if you are doing the exact same thing a week later? Go over it all again.

I apologize for once again taking the fun out of fun. I say all of this not to dissuade you from exploring your sexuality, but since moral panickers are gonna moral panic, I want you to be aware of all possibilities, no matter how rare, so you can be proactive in playing safely. It's no different from discussing different types of birth control and STI prevention options. I'm the boring safety-first auntie and would be hella upset at myself if I didn't share this information and you got caught up in legal trouble that may have been avoidable.

COMMON QUESTIONS ABOUT BDSM

A weird thing happened some years ago that led to the publication of my first zine with Microcosm Publishing, called *BDSM FAQ*. I started getting more and more younger couples coming to my office with questions and concerns about BDSM. Not long-term clients needing to work through complicated issues, but people who wanted to see me once or twice because they were exploring this aspect of their relationship with their partner.

We totally have the movie *Fifty Shades of Grey* to thank for this trend. The books were a crazy-huge success and the first movie was considered #HotAF by many of the people who saw it. But then something else happened. Couples were using *Fifty Shades* role-play in their relationships and feeling . . . well . . . skeeved out. It felt controlling and creepy; not at all the hot and fun experience they had intended. And this makes total sense. *Fifty Shades of Grey* is fantasy, and has little in common with how BDSM works in real life. Mr. Grey, were he a real person, would be a controlling abuser, not the hot and caring dom he is held up to be in the movie.

But a lot of people, including therapists, didn't understand that the story wasn't reflective of how BDSM is practiced in real life. A couple of years after the release of the original *Fifty Shades* movie, a survey of therapists found that one-third of us think

BDSM is bad for relationships. If you are a therapist, please don't be part of this group, ok? Research shows, over and over, that it is simply not true. One study, based in Denmark and Norway, found that when comparing "BDSM" couples and "vanilla" couples, the BDSM couples reported more relationship satisfaction, closeness, and trust between partners because of the vulnerability required to undertake BDSM play.

Other studies have found similar results. A study just of psychological characteristics (versus relationship satisfaction as its own construct) demonstrated that, compared to non-practitioners, BDSM practitioners were less neurotic, were more extraverted, were more open to new experiences, were more conscientious, were less rejection sensitive, and had higher subjective well-being, yet were less "agreeable." So the only "negative" was that they were less agreeable, which means BDSM practitioners are better at standing up for themselves and not doing things they aren't comfortable with . . . yeah, not so much a negative.

All this is to say that, while much of the initial weirdness around *Fifty Shades* has settled down a bit, the importance of the cultural shift towards the acceptance of BDSM has been huge. It's opened up new ways for people to explore their sexual selves and new opportunities for research around how BDSM impacts our mental health in multiple ways, once we stop trying to act like Mr. Grey, that is. And as I mentioned earlier in this book, BDSM is the one domain of kink that isn't gendered around participant interest. Whereas fetishes and many other kinks are generally the domain of (presumably cis) men, BDSM has established all-genders equity. This is because it's such a playful way of engaging with power dynamics and maybe even our shadow selves through fantasy enactment. All of that makes it a very cool and important subject for research.

This chapter covers almost everything I am asked by people who are newer to BDSM play. It isn't intended to be the one and only authoritative BDSM guide, but it should help get you started. I am going to include all the stuff about BDSM that so many were new to and curious about, because it continues to be the kind of information individuals are seeking.

And for the record: If you are really interested in exploring BDSM within the context of cinema, I'm a bigger fan of *Secretary*, starring James Spader and Maggie Gyllenhaal. It's the OG of #HotAF BDSM.

While that movie is queuing up for you, keep reading.

What is BDSM?

As I mentioned in this book's intro, BDSM (also sometimes referred to as S&M) stands for bondage, domination, sadism, and masochism. Depending on who you talk to, the D may stand for discipline instead of domination and the S may stand for submission instead of sadism. Either way, it's a catch-all term for erotic control play.

Let's go a little bit beyond the literal definition.

BDSM has what we call the "Three Cs": consent, control, and communication.

Consent: BDSM is always based on consent for all parties involved. Consent fluctuates and can change and adapt over time. Consent is negotiated ahead of time and throughout the interaction. (If you skipped the consent section in the last chapter, you might want to head back there to learn more details on this.)

Control: BDSM is about control in many different forms, not just the control of one human being by another. The dom also has to be in complete control of themselves at all times in order to respect the boundaries and ensure the safety of their sub.

Communication: BDSM is seriously, seriously, seriously about communication. You have to talk about everything going on before, during, and after the experience. You may consent to something and realize later that you hit a boundary you didn't realize existed. Your interests may change and fluctuate over encounters or periods of time. What makes BDSM healthy is the fact that involved parties are constantly having conversations about what is going on.

Each BDSM interaction should include "straight time" at the end to discuss the experience. Some people even set up contracts for their play time, which I think can provide a lot of legal safety and make everyone involved feel more secure, especially if this is a new thing for you.

Don't freak out though—BDSM can be experimental and light fun . . . not everything has to involve a drama llama of a contract. BDSM is like an onion. Lots of layers. Hopefully, none of them make you cry, though. Unless, of course, that's your thing.

So, BDSM is about sex?

Usually. Though sometimes BDSM is about the mindfuck rather than the act of sex. It's a turn-on, but no erogenous stimulation is taking place. Don't get me wrong—physical release is good. But it may not be the end result in BDSM play.

Ok, so explain to me why this is considered fun?

You know that little kid who spins in circles until they are dizzy? Then they lie down and giggle and watch the world tilt on its axis? And then there's that other little kid sitting in the corner with a pretty complex book, maybe totally past their reading level? But it's fascinating to them, so they're slogging through it because the story is totally making *their* world tilt on *its* axis?

You're feeling me on this, right? Each kid thinks the other kid is making life way too complicated. And they are both correct. What makes the world excellent for THEM, is what makes the world excellent . . . for them.

BDSM is fun for some people because it is. They like setting up situations where power and control interplay with sexual desire and satiation. It makes life fun. Some people aren't interested in that at all. Some people dig it a little bit. Some people are all about BDSM all the time. The world tilts differently for different people.

And sometimes we surprise ourselves and find new things that get us going!

I don't know if I wanna get all that complex. I was thinking maybe a little tying up or something.

I hear ya! Remember how I said BDSM had layers? Another way to think about it is that it exists on a continuum. Kinda like going to the gym. Some people go every day and have serious rock-hard abs. Some go a couple times a week and do a little cardio. Some people only get exercise when reaching for the box of cookies. You can do super pervy with extra kinky sauce or a little vanilla with sprinkles.

Of course, the more you play and the kinkier you get, the more risk is involved (both physically and emotionally) and the more careful you have to be. So no matter what you're planning on, it's all good information to be aware of!

There is a hella lot of lingo swirling around that I don't understand.

IKR?? Just like any subculture, BDSM has its own lingo. Here are a few terms that I get asked about the most.

Age Play – Consensual activities in which at least one participant role-plays being an age other than their actual, chronological age. This term is most often used when one individual is pretending to be younger than the age of consent but is "of age" in reality.

Bondage – The consensual restriction of a partner's movement with one's body or other restraints.

Discipline – Activities in which one person consensually trains another person to act or behave in a particular manner. The root word, from the 1300s, presumed a physicality associated with discipline (lashes with a whip, etc., hence the term being connected so specifically and literally with BDSM).

Dom/Top – You figured this one out already. This is the dominant partner, who is the active controller of the activity in the relationship, the one who is the face of the power play.

Edge Play – Edge play pushes across the boundaries of the Three Cs because it moves into more risk of physical harm, such as erotic asphyxiation. It can be more risky, because you are asking someone to push against boundaries that you have established to see how far you can go. It's considered a form of risk-aware consensual kink (RACK). You are still consenting and you still have an eject button. In edge play you are trusting your partner to take you further than you thought you could go, but still in a healthy, supportive way, and with full respect for your hard boundaries.

Impact Play – The umbrella term for any consensual activity in which you are hitting someone else or being hit with any object (including your own hands).

Munch – This one's not dirty at all actually. A munch is a social gathering, at a restaurant or some other safe environment, for people interested in BDSM to meet other people in the community, ask questions, and see if they want to try it out. You may see a little more leather than you would at a regular table at Denny's, but that's about it.

Safe Words – This is huge. These words are a signal to your partner that you need to stop activities. That you got hurt, physically or emotionally, that a boundary was crossed (maybe one you didn't know existed for yourself), etc. Agree on your word or phrase ahead of time, and never use it unless you mean it. For the record, *no* is a bad safe word. People who engage in edge play (see above) use the word *no* quite often as part of the play without meaning "stop." Pick a word that will not be a part of your play and use that.

Sensory Deprivation – Any situation in which certain human senses are consensually limited to enhance or heighten other senses (like enhancing touch by removing or muffling hearing and vision).

Sub/Bottom – This is the submissive partner who is receiving the action and being controlled. They are the ones with the real power in the relationship, which I'll explain more in a bit.

Switch – Someone who is interested in taking on both Dominant and submissive roles, depending on circumstances. They may sometimes be a dom and sometimes a sub.

How many people actually do this? Or want to?

There are a ton of studies out there. Short version is that about one-third of the population at any given time has experimented with BDSM activities. The vast majority of people have said they have definitely fantasized about it. So there you go, you aren't nearly alone.

So, BDSM is hella hardcore and I'm gonna get the crap beat out of me?

Nope. No pain may be involved at all. It's about power and control. There are many levels to BDSM. It may be a matter of the dominant partner directing all the actions of the submissive one. It may include being tied up with scarves and tickled with a feather. It may mean spankings. It may mean hardcore *needle play*. YMMV. And *it's your choice*.

So, people involved in BDSM are complete weirdos who never have normal sex?

Again, everything exists on a spectrum. Some people have fetishes that all their sexual desires operate through, while some people use BDSM to spice up their otherwise vanilla sex lives. The big question is . . . where on the spectrum are you and your partner(s), and is everyone involved ok with that? For instance, maybe you're seeing someone who can't get off unless they spank you . . . and you like being spanked a lot, but sometimes you just wanna watch Netflix, chill, and have basic missionary sex. It's important to think and talk about all of this.

Yeah, but I heard about this guy who was into BDSM and everyone said he was actually abusing his partner.

I'm sure you have. Abuse gets masked in many different ways. And the BDSM community may be healthier than the general population in several respects, but it still has people in it who need help. Just like there are many amazing men and women who join the city council because they want to serve their community, and then there are the ones who abuse the power and privilege of their position. For the same reasons, there are people who are drawn to BDSM because they are trying to mask abuse, not because they are really into BDSM play.

Now I'm going to share a story (with the author's permission, under the condition of anonymity) that shows that these abuse dynamics do happen in BDSM communities. The author had a very positive experience with BDSM but saw others who did not and wanted to share some of what she saw as a warning to others to make sure they are safe and protected in the community.

A BDSM Story

By Anonymous

*I*n my early 30s, I was searching for something—excitement, something new, something I could learn from. What I found was all of that and, of course, it was on the fringes of our social norms. I have never been a typical, normal kind of person. I have always looked for and felt most comfortable in the out-of-the-ordinary stuff.

What I found was BDSM. I met a man who began to groom me, mold me into a submissive. It was a humbling experience, considering that I have never been in that kind of position. I have always been the dominant personality in my relationships. This relationship was as intimate as any romantic relationship; he got to know me in a way that I had not even explored myself.

When we met, he had 15 years of experience, and had a mentor. He slowly introduced me into the lifestyle, giving me the language to use, defining behaviors, and defining expectations. While he did his part of educating me, he also encouraged me to educate myself about the lifestyle.

During my training, I got to meet some good people. I would attend BDSM group meetings, meet other dominants and submissives, attend submissive-specific meet-and-greets, and view online profiles of other submissives and their alleged daily lives. I also was encouraged to learn what it meant to be a dominant. All of the education I obtained was at the encouragement of my dominant. He would often tell me that I needed to know what was out there; I needed to know how far I would go.

In the lifestyle, you learn the terminology and you learn the basic manners and behaviors of both dominant and submissive.

Each Master is different, with differing levels of education and experience. There are those who are both dominant and submissive. Some dominants have families of submissives—and some submissives have multiple Masters. There are polyamorous families. It is a very diverse population, even within the small subculture that it is.

During my year and a half in the lifestyle, I got to meet many other submissives and hear their stories. What I heard was horrifying. I heard stories of abuse, rape, lies, and manipulation. I heard of submissives that had childhood trauma and it was being lived out in their kinky relationship. I heard of Masters who were abusing submissives and calling it "being a dominant."

I heard of dominants dropping submissives because, as a Master, they had not been pleased to their fullest. I heard of Masters who would push limits. Limits that were meant to be static.

My own Master was the opposite of these horrifying stories. He was compassionate, patient, and understanding and wanted me to be educated about both the lifestyle and my limits. He wanted me to make healthy choices. But he would not attend community/lifestyle meetings—he knew what was out there and no longer agreed with it. He believed in the lifestyle, but he also believed that many "Dominants" were nothing more than abusers who had found a willing victim.

I would often reflect on this while hearing those submissives' stories and ask if it was what they really wanted. They would often hesitate and say, "Not all of it, but it comes with being a submissive." They, too, had been groomed, but they had been groomed by an abuser to believe that their experience in the lifestyle was what it was all about.

Many times, I would leave meetings feeling worried about those submissives. I worried that they would be hurt even more than what they had already experienced.

As I continued to learn from various sources—my Master, the other submissives, community members, and online resources—I began to see a fine line between those who I considered true dominants and opportunistic predators.

I learned that while I was labeled the submissive, I actually held quite a bit of power. My Master was given permission, by me, to behave and formulate expectations that I had guided. I, after all, would be enduring the pleasures of someone else. My being would be defined by someone else when I was with him. This was not taken lightly by my Master or myself.

I did not realize it at the time, but he was making sure I was educated to give my consent. I was able to set soft limits and hard limits that he would respect. Soft limits are boundaries that can be manipulated or pushed, while hard limits are static and are not allowed to be manipulated. We would spend hours talking about the things we each liked and the things I was willing to do and not do. He would allow me to set soft limits while I determined if it would remain soft or become a hard limit. He would explain that as we built trust, my soft and hard limits would begin to dissolve. All this time, he would seek my consent to move forward, stopping when necessary.

He would often ask if I was ok, or if I was ready, before pushing boundaries for the first time. If I displayed any hesitancy, he would stop. He was patient and would wait or stop altogether.

He was compassionate while we discussed my fears and my concerns. I was never made to feel less-than and I was never made to feel guilt.

Looking back, I realize how different my experience was from that of some of the other submissives. I was able to feel in control of myself, I gave my consent at every new endeavor. In educating myself on the idea of consent, I learned about CREST: consent, respect, equality, safety, and trust. In the lifestyle, a dominant allegedly has all the power, and the submissive serves the dominant. It seems counterintuitive to think that we are equal, but in my experience, it worked that way. He was able to combine all these healthy factors into our BDSM relationship. I always felt respected, I felt safe, and I trusted my Master. I felt equal in the ability to say no when I wanted to, knowing that he would take what I said and felt into consideration—like in any relationship.

This was so different from what I was hearing from some of the other submissives. They would often complain that they felt used by their Master. They would relay stories of how their hard limits had been ignored and they would be left feeling guilty for being upset, or shamed for not being a good submissive. I would try to ask about their trust-building process, but would get a response filled with defensiveness, often claiming that I was too new to the community to understand.

They would joke of certain Masters that had a high turnover of submissives. This left me feeling disheartened by the lifestyle, disillusioned about being a part of the community, and coming around to my Master's view of the community.

While not all of the submissives I met struggled with these issues, I found enough in the community to be worried about people's safety. Worried that these women and men were being either victimized or revictimized, reliving their childhood traumas, and getting caught in an unhealthy cycle.

This experience helped me to learn quite a bit about myself and life. I learned that one can learn how to be a dominant personality. Sometimes it's an act, and that's ok. Being a dominant personality requires patience, compassion, honesty, and an understanding that people have limitations, and that needs to be respected. I learned that our childhoods haunt us, and if we are not careful, our pasts will find a way to manifest in our daily lives.

I left that lifestyle with all these lessons under my belt, and they continue to exist with me today. I have always been a leader, but until I learned from my Master I led with aggression, fear, and lies. My childhood traumas impact me on occasion, and I have gained the insight to address it when I notice it. I am able to be a leader with compassion, understanding, and patience. I am respectful of people's limitations.

In choosing to leave the lifestyle, I hoped to define my experience by learning what I could. I hoped to frame this experience to help me be a better human being.

If you are looking for a Dominant partner, talk to other people you trust in the community and look for warning signs. Do they go through a lot of subs pretty quickly? Do they push past clearly established boundaries that you have set? Are they altered with drugs and alcohol past the point of self-control? Are they simply stating their expectations and commanding you to follow through, rather than giving you homework to educate you about your role and theirs? Do they just plain make you feel unsafe? You don't have to take that.

If you are looking for a submissive partner, look for someone who has clear boundaries and communicates them and takes responsibility for themselves in the relationship.

What about these subs with a tough past? Aren't there people out there who are using BDSM to relive their trauma over and over?

Not usually (though as we've shown throughout the book and especially in the personal story above, it can happen). The rate of individuals with a trauma history in the BDSM community is no higher than in the general population. If you do have a trauma history, BDSM actually has the potential to be very healing (but only if it's practiced the right way, as illustrated by our anonymous story). Being a submissive in a BDSM relationship does not mean you are giving up all control. In fact, it is the polar opposite. The sub in a BDSM relationship is the one with all the power. The dom has to be in complete control of themselves in order to ensure that boundaries are not crossed, that their sub is always safe, and that they can immediately stop if the safe word is utilized. That is a lot of power. And the sub has most of it.

If you are an abuse survivor, the main question to ask yourself about your BDSM relationship is: Do you feel secure and in control of the experience? If the answer is no or not sure, seeing a trauma-trained therapist to help you figure some of that out might make a lot of sense.

Is everyone who is into BDSM into swinging/polyamory/ the lifestyle?

Nope. But you will see a lot of overlap. The reason is that when you are in the practice of communicating your wants and needs to a partner, there will be things you may be interested in that they are not. You may end up negotiating in order to have that need met elsewhere.

Just like BDSM, it's negotiated, always. Some worry that swinging is cheating, but cheating is about the lie, not the act. Many people in the BDSM community have other partners for certain activities, while many others are happily monogamous. If you become involved in the community but want to remain monogamous, that will be respected.

How do you stay safe with all this risky stuff going on?

You stay safe by minimizing the risks and learning what you are doing before you start. And you always have an escape hatch, like a safe word. Reading and talking to others in the community is extremely beneficial for safety if you are going beyond very basic things.

For example, if your interest is tying up, you don't want to knot the rope (or scarves, or whatever you are using), since a knot can easily cut off circulation and be difficult to untie in a hurry. There are resources to help you learn tying techniques that protect your sub partner.

While tied up, you need to be able to maintain constant communication about your ability to still maintain circulation. If you struggle to notice circulation issues in yourself (for example, if you are diabetic and have neuropathy), your dom partner may ask you to push up against their hand to show that you aren't numb. If you aren't able to, or otherwise complain that you are losing sensation, your dom partner needs to have a sharp cutting implement available to immediately cut you free.

You can see how the more complicated you get, the more careful you have to be. And that's a good thing.

Now let's go a little deeper into some acronyms we talked about in the last chapter. The acronym embraced within much of the kink community, proposed by Gary Switch of *Prometheus* magazine in 1999, is RACK (risk-aware consensual kink), which was a replacement to the '80s term SSC (safe, sane, and consensual). You may be curious about the change-over, so here's the tea.

Nothing is safe. Not really. We want to have safer sex as much as we want to have safer sword fighting. Or even just safer driving to work and cooking dinner on a hot stove. And while both terms center consensuality, RACK changes the spirit of play by reminding us that everything is risky. And being risk-aware means everyone involved knows which risks we may be taking and how we will handle ourselves if things go sideways. Being risk-aware means we continue to seek out more education and practice and feedback so we build our expertise around increasing the safety of whatever fun, sexy play we enjoy.

However, the National Coalition for Sexual Freedom warns that there are potential legal problems with the use of the term. If a scene architect uses the term *RACK* in pre-scene planning, the concern is that they are acknowledging risk of harm in a way that creates legal liability for them if something does go wrong. If that is your concern (and it's a legit concern!), another framework you may prefer to utilize is PRICK (personal responsibility, informed, consensual kink). While similar to RACK, PRICK centers the responsibility and consequences of risky behavior upon the person taking the risk in consensual exchanges. Also? PRICK is funnier than RACK. And I'm all for the types of jokes that make my inner 12-year-old laugh her ass off.

To illustrate what PRICK looks like in practice, let's use our bondage example again. Agreeing on safe words and safe gestures isn't enough. What if you lose circulation? What if you have some form of neuropathy and maybe can't always tell that's what's happening? A discussion about that would be had, and something to help keep you safer would be put into place. So if, say, your arms are tied and elevated over your head, your play partner could put their hand just over yours and tell you to push your hand up into theirs. And if you could not do so, they would cut the rope.

But the PRICK acronym has also gotten pushback. This includes the argument that if you are new to a certain activity, you can't be completely informed, especially regarding the emotional response you might have. The language around this stuff is always evolving, and not everyone is going to agree on it.

Ok, we communicated and negotiated and all that stuff you said to try, and we want to move forward. How do we get started? Do I just start tying my partner up or what?

If you have a willing partner, and you just want to go home and start the tying, go for it . . . just be safe! Check out your local toy store, find stuff that interests you, and try a few things out. But keep in mind that part of the reason that BDSM has a big community is not just to find partners (or find secondary partners) but to support each other, learn from each other, and help other people practice safely. If you are concerned about any of that, getting to know others in the community can be helpful. Besides attending a munch, you can check out other events (especially conferences and classes!) and participate at your level of comfort. Ask questions, be safe!

If you want to *find* a willing partner, the aforementioned FetLife website is your best bet. If you have a job where your footprints online may be an issue, a traditional dating site that includes many people who aren't as traditional is a better bet. You will still definitely see profiles for individuals who are interested in the same thing you are. When you're looking for a partner, be clear about your boundaries and watch out for the red and yellow flags.

What if I'm looking for the BDSM community in my area and I don't want a digital footprint from bopping around online?

If you would rather keep everything IRL, use social media and other sites like Meetup to look for in-person events, like an upcoming munch or info about other events. You can browse in private mode and run a VPN and a tunnel if you want to mitigate your digital footprint in your searches. Larger areas have clubs (in San Antonio we have a couple at any given time, on top of the private parties) and many smaller areas still have events (private parties, pop-up events, etc.) organized online through Meetup, FetLife, and the like.

Just a thought: If you are looking online, use an email that you don't use for anything else, FFS. If you are really concerned about keeping this part of your life private, you may want to use a burner phone number for communications, one that you don't tie to your regular social media accounts and the like.

***What if I just want to try some stuff out but don't want
to take out a second mortgage or meet a bunch of
people who own way more leather than I'm interested in
owning? No munches, no rope . . . just a little sumpin-
sumpin new?***

Roll with that! If the majority of people out there have fantasized
about BDSM at one point or another . . . chances are most of
them weren't thinking about how they would like to turn their
rec room into a dungeon. A lot of BDSM play is way low risk.
For example, there are many kinds of handcuffs that the sub can
release themselves from easily, meaning they are never really out
of control of the situation. This goes back to a previous question.
Go check out a local toy store and find some things that interest
you, bring them home, and start playing. If you are at a place or
get to a place where you want to go a little deeper, look at maybe
connecting to the community for some support.

***Speaking of just trying some stuff out . . . I am interested
in some things, but not other things. That gonna be a
problem?***

Not even. The great thing about the BDSM community is the
strong respect for consent. Rejection of an offer is just that:
Rejection of an offer. Not of the person. There may be some
things you are interested in on some days and not others.
There may be some things you never want to do. It may be that
sometimes you really want to try something and then realize you
had a boundary triggered and need to stop. All of this is ok.

It's important to remember that this goes both ways. A
rejection of your offer is not a rejection of you. Clearly you are
awesome, so do your best not to take it personally.

My partner wants to do this, but I have zero interest.

Congratulations, you are grown. This means you are responsible for your bills, but on the upside you have complete authority over your own body and what you do with it. You don't have to do any of this if you aren't comfortable. I'm sure this is a point of contention in the relationship, one that a good, kink-friendly counselor can help you navigate.

Please be aware that this chapter is *information* about BDSM. It is NOT a manifesto. It is not my job to insist you like BDSM, just to answer some of the questions I often get. I appreciate you learning more and I hope your partner does as well. I hope that reading this can help start a new conversation with your partner about how to better navigate your relationship. And use a website like the Kink Aware Professionals (KAP) listings to find a counselor in your area who will support your conversations.

Anything else?

Of course there is tons more about BDSM out there, and there are bunches of people whose careers are spent teaching and writing about this. This info is intended not to replace any of their work, but to answer some of the basic questions and normalize a part of sexual expression that is actually completely, legitimately, totally normal.

Whether you want to be blindfolded or you fantasize about being suspended upside down, you're not the least bit weird for that. BDSM is exactly what you make it . . . and it can be fun and fulfilling and enjoyable if navigated with communication and respect. Enjoy yourself!

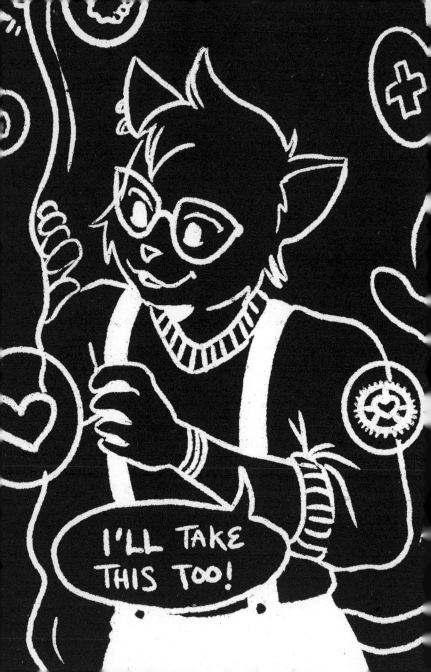

OTHER WAYS TO GET YOUR KINK ON

So maybe BDSM isn't your thing. Or maybe it *is* your thing, but you also have other things that you want to explore. In this chapter, we'll go over some tips for engaging in a bunch of different types of kink besides BDSM (though plenty of the info in this chapter can also apply to BDSM—there's a lot of overlap). Because ropes and domination are great and all, but there's a whole lot of other stuff out there too.

Fantasy and Role-Play Exist and They're Fun

While BDSM can definitely have a fantasy or role-play component (and really you could argue that all BDSM is a form of role-play), you can also engage in fantasy and role-play without having the power-differential component of BDSM.

To be honest, I hadn't really thought about this being its own separate entity until a good number of my gender-nonconforming clients talked about their use of role-play in sexual intimacy. If people trust me enough to talk about that stuff, I totally need to listen. And I found that, as with BDSM, the experience can be profoundly healing when approached in the right way. So let's address a few points.

Fantasy Is Not Reality

About 75% of our sexual fantasies are about sexual activities that we have already established that we are engaged in or intend to engage in. Whatever our definition of "normal" sex may be. Which means the other 25% are about things that have some level of intrigue for us but aren't something we necessarily want to try out.

So much of what we fantasize about does not reflect our true interests. I've had clients tell me, with great horror, how they told their partner about a fantasy they had. But when their partner went to the trouble of trying to fulfill it for them, my clients were embarrassed to find that they actually had no real interest.

When studying both heterosexual and homosexual men, Masters and Johnson found that both groups fantasized about having sex with a person who was not the gender they were typically attracted to. That was as high on the list as BDSM fantasies, group-sex fantasies, and all of the other common fantasies that people experience. And the fact that people had these fantasies didn't invalidate their sexual orientation or mean that they wanted to engage in these activities for real.

The checklist I use with clients about sexual activities has four options: yes, no, I don't know, and fantasy only. Being intrigued by an idea or turned on by it isn't the same thing as being interested in trying it out in real life.

Fantasy Is Not Obsession

A 2015 study found that up to 62% of women had experienced rape fantasies. Do 62% of women secretly harbor a desire to be raped? Maybe some losers in 4chan-type places think so, but I seriously doubt it. The researcher looked at how often the fantasy occurred . . . and it wasn't often. Once a week, maybe once a month. And it wasn't tied to the idea of not having to take responsibility for a sexual encounter; instead, it was tied to younger generations (millennials and Zers) being experientially open and fantasy allowing them to express that without experiencing actual violation.

Role-Play Can Allow an Authentic Identity to Be Present

In my practice, I've seen a huge jump in clients who are into sexual role-play. As a Gen Xer, I definitely knew about furry parties and the like, but the internet has made it so much easier to find people with similar interests and engage in sex with them, setting up elaborate stories and settings in which they can enact certain roles that would otherwise be impossible.

I've seen this to be especially true of my clients who are trans or otherwise gender nonconforming. If you feel uncomfortable in your physical presentation, role-playing as someone else allows you a new level of freedom. Many younger clients told me that non-sexual role-playing games brought their first awareness of their gender identity, and that starting in puberty they found themselves picking characters of their authentic gender instead of their birth-assigned gender.

A lot of people are just big fans of certain characters and really enjoy cosplay. Bringing that cosplay into their sexual relationships simply enhances the experience . . . you don't need to hate your body in order to enjoy being someone else now and then!

Things to Watch Out For

While I am totally the queen of "you do you and let your freak flag fly," sexual fantasy and role-play can end up being problematic. Just like anything else fun, right? Here are some warning signs:

1. Just like with sex and porn misusage, if the fantasy and role-play take the place of real engagement with other human beings, there might be a problem.

2. If your fantasies do move into perseveration territory, meaning they occupy your thoughts and you feel impulses to act on things you know are wrong or find disturbing, that could be a problem too.

3. If your partners in role-play are violating your boundaries under the guise, especially online, that it isn't real sex, that's not ok. It's important to set and keep boundaries (in character or out) that protect you from being hurt. (Tip from a gamer friend: If you don't want to have a conversation about why you're leaving, announce that you are having connection issues and then log out.)

If you are noticing patterns of problem behavior in yourself, find a sex-positive, kink-aware professional to work with on developing better usage strategies and coping skills.

Toys and Other Gear

When you start to get kinky, there's often equipment involved. Sex toys can be anything you use to enhance your sex life that isn't your body or a partner's body. Like vibrators, masturbation sleeves, rope for BDSM play, and Ben Wa balls. But also fly swatters, grapefruit, and paracord. Yes, anything. Cement mixer? Sure, if you're brave enough. They may be something fun to play with or an adaptation that allows you to experience a healthy sex life (whether partnered or solo) that you wouldn't be able to experience otherwise. Even people who don't need toys for physical functioning can get a lot of enjoyment out of adding a little spice to their life. Using them isn't a sign of failure, perversion, or inability to function independently. Saying sex without sex toys is better than sex with sex toys is as goofy as saying the only right sexual position is the missionary position. And if you've made it this far into this book, you're probably way past the point of believing that.

Types of Sex Toys

Here are the main (and far from all-inclusive) categories of toys that you might encounter:

Vibrators: Today, the biggest share of the sex toy market goes toward toys that vibrate. These toys can be used internally or externally, and the vibration gives you lots of sensory stimulus. Beyond what you might traditionally think of as a vibrator, there are also vibrating cock rings, vibrating anal plugs, vibrating nipple clamps, and more. Even the traditional, phallic-shaped vibrator is not just for use on vulvas—many find the vibrations to be pleasurable when held against their other erogenous zones.

Insertables: This includes things you can put inside yourself. You know. Up the vagina, up the booty hole. In the mouth. Butt plugs, dildos, etc. Anything that allows you the sensation of being filled up and enjoying the pleasure of something connecting to your body on the inside.

Strokers: These are used to stroke the outside of whatever genitalia you're working with. For instance, the Fleshlight for an individual with a penis or a clit stroker for someone with a vulva. Another great example of the market catching up to the need is strokers designed specifically to allow trans men the stroking sensation that cis men enjoy, while taking into account that, if on testosterone, they often have larger genitalia than most cis women.

Restraints: Ropes! Blindfolds! Gags! These next several categories will lead us back into BDSM territory, but hey, I said there'd be overlap. Restraints allow you to play with power safely when good trust and boundaries are established. You can also get super elaborate and fancy with restraints and create some gorgeous aesthetics, whether you were an Eagle Scout or not.

Clamps: Stuff that pinches your skin for localized sensation. Nipples are popular, but people will clamp all kinds of body parts. While restraints may or may not be used to produce pain, clamps generally are. Why does it feel so good to have our skin pinched in these situations? Pain and pleasure share the same neurobiology, and we get a huge endorphin burst!

Floggers: Whips, paddles, anything to hit, spank, or provide a heavier, stronger skin impact. Like clamps or restraints, floggers can produce pain without you having to wear out your hands or your partner's hands.

Sensory toys: If you're looking for extra sensations or stimulation, the options out there are vaster than you may realize. In addition to vibrators, there are many other sex toys designed to enhance your sensory experience. Some use textures (velvet, fur, feathers, leather, wood, metal), some use temperature changes (hot or cold), some are designed to take away your sense of control in one area to enhance your enjoyment of another (e.g., blindfolds, noise-canceling headphones), and, of course, many vibrate to provide additional oomph.

Lubes, oils, and creams: Another huge part of the sex toy market. Lubricants are designed to facilitate ease of movement over the skin in partnered or unpartnered activity. There are wet lubricants (typically water- or silicone-based) and dry lubricants (such as graphite-based) that add to the comfort of the sexual experience. Many creams are designed to either enhance sensation (as when cinnamon is used for tingling) or dampen sensation to lengthen time engaged in sexual activity. Many creams are also flavored, which can help facilitate comfort with oral activity. Oils are often a combination of lubes and creams to provide more ease of movement, plus other ingredients to help with sensation.

Supports: Swings, pillows, wedges, grab bars, anything that helps you get into the position you're wanting. The support may be medically necessary, helpful but not necessary, or purely for getting a different sensory experience.

As you explore, you'll see there are plenty of options that don't neatly fit into any category on this list. Sorry about that . . . the industry is amazing and coming up with new items on the regular, and more and more of them are adaptable to gender variations and mobility issues. Suffice to say there is a lot of fun stuff out there designed to enhance your sexual experience, no matter how kinky you want to get. And not everything is designed specifically to provide direct stimulation to your naughty bits.

Where to Find Sex Toys and Supplies

As you embark on your kinky odyssey, consider making a trip to the "adult novelty store," aka the sex toy store. Sex toys are available both online and in brick-and-mortar stores in most communities. And the stores are not dirty, dark, back-alley places filled with creepy guys in trench coats anymore. They are clean, well lit, and professionally managed. It's like going to Target, except with a display of French ticklers.

And an increasing number of these stores are specifically feminist, owned and staffed by women, trans people, and nonbinary people, which makes for a whole different experience.

Safety and Cleaning

Ok, boring sex educator making safety suggestions again. There really is a good safety benefit to using barrier methods (like condoms or dams) on any objects that you use internally or that come into contact with soft tissues and mucous membranes. I know, I know . . . the whole point of having toys is so that you *don't* have to use barrier methods to prevent pregnancy and STIs. But while a toy won't get you pregnant, you can still pass on STIs (and run-of-the-mill bacterial infections, which in this case are *still* sexually transmitted) or spread them to other parts of your body through toys that were not properly cleaned. Or you can reinfect yourself with something that's already been treated. Any toys that are porous can also become bacteria-harboring grub monsters (blech). So use barrier methods, even with toys, and take good care of your goodies by following the cleaning tips below.

Don't use a perfumed soap, the ingredients used for scent can irritate your skin. Dr. Bronner's soap is great stuff and comes unscented for sensitive folx. A good-quality antibacterial soap is best. You want to wipe them down, not dunk them (unless they are a waterproof toy, in which case, dunk away).

Don't put your rubber- and plastic-type toys in the dishwasher, you can totally melt them. Other than glass toys or stainless steel, you wanna stay away from the dishwasher.

Leather – Wipe down with soap and water or use a special leather cleaner. If the leather comes in contact with bodily fluids, you can disinfect it by wiping it down with a 70% isopropyl rubbing alcohol solution.

Glass – Wash with soap and water.

Rubber – if it's something that is going to be inserted, use a condom or dam . . . rubber is super porous, so it holds bacterial grubbies way too well. Also? Rubber can contain phthalate, which is not something you want seeping into your never-minds (if you wouldn't eat it, don't stick it up anywhere, either).

Silicone – Wash with soap and water.

Stainless steel – Wash with soap and water. If you want to be extra about it, stainless steel can go in the dishwasher or can be soaked in a solution of 10:1 water and bleach for 10 minutes.

Vinyl and Cyberskin – These are very porous materials that are pretty fragile. These are best washed in warm water and left to air dry. They can get sticky easily, so dusting them with cornstarch is also a good idea (fun fact: corn starch doesn't clump up).

Nylon (paracord is made of nylon, FYI) – Can be washed in the washing machine or by hand with soap and water. You can also remove odor from nylon by soaking it in a solution of water and baking soda.

Fabrics – Wash all fabric as you would fabric you are wearing on your body. Cotton, polyester, and bamboo and the like do fine in a washing machine, silks and wools do better dry cleaned or gently hand washed if you feel confident in managing these materials. Fabric ropes need to be left to air dry in coils and stretched occasionally during the drying period so they don't kink up (you are already kinky enough, right, playa?).

Hemp – Hemp can be machine washed on gentle and air dried (it will take two to five days to dry completely, so plan accordingly). If you are washing hemp rope, you will want to knot it and place it in a pillow case before washing (there are lots of videos online with knotting techniques to prepare rope for washing). Hemp rope can be re-oiled (baby oil or jojoba oil are good) after drying.

Group Sex, Swingers, and Sex Clubs

There is a decent-sized overlap between consensual non-monogamy and kink. It is hopefully obvious that this is not a requirement, but many people find that the play-forward part of consensual non-monogamy fits very well into their kink lifestyle. Think sex parties, sex clubs, swinging events, and similar activities that may not lead to longer-term relationships. Funsies stuff. Clubs and parties offer a great outlet for things like voyeurism (meaning you like to watch others) and exhibitionism (meaning you like to be watched). And some of them focus only on the kink scenes with no actual sex. In recent years I've seen some of the sexy-but-not-sexual play show up in other adjacent scenes, which is a great idea. One example is fet fashion shows with a separate spanking room for interested guests.

If you are curious about this scene, but feeling a bit overwhelmed and nervous about the idea, let's get you started. First of all, the aforementioned websites FetLife and Meetup are good starting points for finding spots in your area. And if you have a seasoned kinkster available, ask them about dress code, rules, and expectations. There may be subtleties to your local scene that will inform your decision making. This information should be provided at any event you attend, but feeling prepared ahead of time can go a long way toward alleviating your nerves.

Some other points to consider:

1. This may be a place for your enjoyment, but for other people it is where they work. Respect employees and volunteers, like the room safety proctors. Don't be a dick to people doing their jobs, enforcing rules, etc.

2. These environments are high-consent areas, or at least they fucking should be. If they aren't, feel free to report it or dip on out of there. So for example, if you are watching some activities and you get invited to join, but you aren't interested? Just say, "No thank you, I'm enjoying watching!"

3. That being said, most people will be delighted if you take initiative in propositioning them. And it's ok to be disappointed if someone tells you "no thank you," but don't get butthurt. It takes the fun out of fun. It's also totally fine to just chat with people. You'll find them generally friendly if they are not . . . busy with other activities at the moment. Say hi and introduce yourself. You don't even have to use your real name if you're worried about it, you can have a scene name that people will use and respect (also pretty common).

4. Respect people's privacy, including your own. It's totally fine to not share anything you don't want to share . . . and that is often respected way more than lying about yourself. And Vegas rules apply. You saw a local county judge at the club? Leave them alone, they aren't doing anything wrong and deserve their freedom of expression and privacy as much as you do. I know a lot of kinksters who are well known to their larger community, but only the kink community knows they're kinky. And that's how it should be.

5. Don't think you're starting a relationship with someone. The scene is just the scene, more often than not. And you may see the same person on other occasions and

never play with them again. It's totally fine on anyone's end to not pursue further contact.

Kinky, Ethical Porn

So hopefully we are on the same page about porn being just another facet of human culture, with both good and bad qualities, *just like everything else*. Porn can be a fantastic way to explore your desires, either solo or with a partner. You can engage in fantasy, role-play, exploring what you find sexually stimulating, and the like. If you are newer to porn viewing, or you've tried before but found some of what you saw to be discomfiting, you might find the experience far different if you actively seek out ethical porn (which is also sometimes referred to as fair trade porn or feminist porn).

You are far more likely to see a wider variety of human bodies (age, size, etc.) and storylines that focus on far more than getting to the money shot. Additionally, these filmmakers are historically far more respectful of the erotic performers they have hired in these roles. Individuals are paid in accordance with their worth and work, and they are far less likely to end up in dangerous situations as employees. And I don't have to tell you that you absolutely should be paying for your porn, right? Whatever you are watching was the end result of several people's jobs. And we respect and value people's labor by paying them what they are worth.

If you do a search for "ethical porn" or one of those other search terms used to define this kind of work, you will find several articles reviewing the companies that endeavor to make porn that is respectful, safe, and still very sexy . . . and this includes companies that focus specifically on kink topics, scenes, and storylines.

Other Sexy Media

If porn feels out of your comfort zone, or is less interesting to you in general, there are plenty of other options out there in this domain. We're talking erotica, sexy art (remember when Tumblr was full of it?), and fan fiction. (Cuz if you are into *Doctor Who* and needle play? Why not find some fanfic that combines both of your favorite topics? If Meco could release Star Wars Disco in 1977, you are allowed whatever weird mash-up makes your pervy little heart happy.) These can all be fun additions to your sexytimes, whether partnered or solo.

Fifty Shades of Grey may be a shit representation of how BDSM actually works, but it was extremely popular anyway . . . because humans just love our smutty smut. It's a good way to explore our kinks, plus the structures we put in place around them. The smuttier books I've read in the past have gotten increasingly good at bringing consent and differential desires and all of those other useful topics into their storylines. And anything you aren't interested in can be easily skimmed over.

If you take in more through audial means, you can find lots and lots of these materials available as MP3s and other sound files. Just don't get so hot and bothered you accidentally smash your bike into a tree out of distraction.

Sex Work and Erotic Performance

Adjacent to porn is sex work and other erotic performance work. I'm categorizing it differently from porn, since porn is generally created for more than one or two viewers, and it's a static item that remains re-viewable, downloadable, and the like. This is different from paying someone directly (or exchanging goods and other services) for them to provide you a titillating experience. This could take the form of camming, chaturbating, dancing, stripping, acting in a kink scene with you, and . . . of course . . . having some kind of sexual exchange either with you or in front of you. Depending on where you live, some or all of these activities may not be legal. It will come as no surprise that I disagree with this stance, and have a pretty large "we need to decriminalize sex work" soap box that I have been known to drag out on many occasions. That's a conversation for a different venue, so I won't rail on about it. For our purposes here, I'll just say that while I think this is an incredibly useful option for many people from all walks of life, there may be consequences both legal and social. So bear this in mind, do your due diligence, and mitigate risk.

And this is another place where connecting to the larger kink community in your area may be of benefit. They can offer safe(r) suggestions if you do the cost analysis around potential legal or social ramifications and determine it's worth it. For example, community members might be able to connect you with a professional dom who is discreet and kind versus someone you found listed in the back of the free weekly paper who may or may not be either of those things.

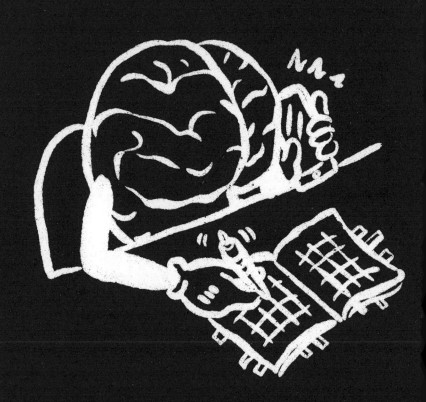

DEAR AUNTIE FAITH, I'M A PERV AND I HAVE QUESTIONS

S ometimes as I'm writing my books, I like to put out a call for questions that it might be helpful to answer. And y'all, being awesome, ask such good questions that instead of folding them all into the text, I often like to answer them directly, like a ratchet Ann Landers or something. And the same thing happened again with this book.

A few of your questions could be answered nicely in the main text, but there were plenty more great questions that I wanted to take the time to answer individually. And they're fun,[8] so let's get to it.

Hey Auntie!

What does non-sexual kink look like?

Hi there, nibling!

I got more than one question about kinks that are "non-sexual." In both cases, I didn't have any information on what the kink is, how it is engaged in, or what role it plays in the participant's happiness and enjoyment. Which makes it really hard to answer this question.

---

8 And I miss writing my sex advice column for a now-defunct magazine! So if anyone wants to hire me to write the sex advice column for their not-defunct publication, please holler at your girl!

Because as you see from all the definitions in this book, kink is defined and operationalized as a behavior that exists for sexual excitement and gratification. Which then means there is no such thing as a non-sexual kink, as far as that definition is concerned. But that's just a definition, and it doesn't invalidate anyone's experience of themselves. Which is also why I say I wish I had more information about your particular situation.

I am guessing wildly here, but I'm thinking you are speaking about something that other people think of as a sexual kink, but it isn't sexual for you (or whomever you are asking on behalf of). Like wearing a rubber catsuit and walking around whipping people or whatever. If that's the case, first of all I'd say, "Fuck yeah . . . do the thing you like and please only whip consenting whipees," and I would also say it's entirely ok to like something that's considered sexual for non-sexual reasons. Maybe it helps you feel playful. Maybe it helps you feel powerful.

Maybe you like engaging in the world from this space for any number of non-sexual reasons. And if that's the case, that's also utterly fine and even wonderful. You don't owe an explanation to anyone about your own business, but if you ever are trying to share information about your likes and preferences, you can say just that. "I like [XYZ thing]. Most people think of it as a kink but for me it's about [ABC reasons]." You're allowed to like what you like for whatever reasons, I promise.

Auntie

Hi Auntie,

How do I deal with accepting my kink that is more extreme than most kinks? The most difficult part is seeing what many kinky people around parts of the internet write about it: "I'm not one to kink shame, but for scat/vomit/

abdl/cnc/other fetishes that are considered 'taboo' even by fetishist standards, I'll make an exception . . ."

Hi there, nibling!

Doesn't that just beat all? Being judged by the same people that are already being judged by greater society. This is such human nature, very similar in my mind to bi/pan folks being told to just "pick a team already!" Sometimes people are determined to put you in an "ew, gross" category of sorts. Or, to invoke the late Michael Aday (best known to my generation as Meat Loaf) . . . they will do anything for love, but they won't do THAT.

Honestly, as a grumpy old(er) lady, my advice would be not to worry about what other people think, if that's affecting your enjoyment of your own body and life. It sounds like maybe you have been struggling with some self-recrimination in this regard. And it can be important to remind yourself how your engagement in your kink is as safe as possible in all the different ways discussed throughout this book. And considerate. And respectful. And consensual. And to also have an answer ready to go when people make stank face about what you like. You may want to mildly remind people that it's important that we respect that people like what they like. While it is our human nature to judge others, we can keep those judgments to ourselves when someone else's behavior isn't impacting us in the least. That kind of stuff. Argument-killer statements.

Now there may be some people who do have a genuine curiosity and want to better understand you. And if they are important enough people in your life, you may want to engage more with them. So think about what you are willing to discuss and what is off the table. Maybe you share how you are considerate and safer, maybe you share a little of what you like about your particular kink. But you don't have to share everything all the time. It's ok to say there are aspects of your experience that you don't want to share.

Here's the thing. There is a huge difference between privacy and secrecy. Secrecy is about something remaining intentionally hidden and contained. Privacy is the space in which you remain unobserved by outsiders. Closing the bathroom door is about privacy, not secrecy, right? We know you're poopin' or something in there . . . we don't need to be involved. You aren't keeping secrets, you're just setting a boundary of privacy.

Auntie

Dear Auntie,

I like to act like a virgin sometimes and encourage my husband to "teach me" what he likes, but I'm worried it's problematic that I'm portraying a young girl, even in the privacy of our own home. It's my kink maybe even more than his, and I never hint at being underage, but even a veiled reference makes me worry I'm crossing an ethical line—should I reconsider my go-to or dig deeper to see if there's an underlying issue here?

Dear nibling,

There are at least two really common kink themes in your dynamic: age play and power play. It seems like the age play part is the part that you are a little worried about. But I've found (and researchers and other individuals in the scene agree) that the age play is just another expression of power play.

And that is the essence of BDSM scenes, right? It's fun to change up power dynamics in a relationship. To put someone else safely in charge of us. It's relaxing to not have to make any of the decisions about a situation, but to know the decisions being made for you will be fun and non-harmful. And it sounds like this is something you both enjoy, so that's awesome.

The other part of your letter I want to respond to is the idea that maybe you need to "dig deeper" to see if there is any underlying trauma response going on. There have been many unfortunate eras of mental health treatments that we now know were shady and unhelpful. The "repressed memories" era is definitely one of them. Brains don't like uncertainty and can mix and match vague memories to confabulate stories that never happened. We've seen this with some techniques in particular, like hypnotherapy. And I say this as someone who practices hypnotherapy and has found it to be a useful therapeutic tool. But I am also very, very, VERY careful not to prod people in certain directions, not to ask them to recover portions of their lives while under hypnosis, etc. It is incredibly easy to build false memories.

I've found that most of the childhood memories people do discuss in these therapeutic contexts are ones that they did already remember. Things that they had worked to not think about so much, maybe. Things they had shoved aside in order to function. Things they didn't remember very well, so they were vague and confusing and disquieting. In which case we recognize that something bad likely happened but that reaching for the particulars isn't going to get us far, so we focus on dealing with the present outfall of trauma responses (because a trauma narrative is not necessary to trauma healing).

So I am guessing that if something had happened to you, you'd have some notion of it. And your interest in this particular scene would feel like something you were compelled to enact and reenact, and it doesn't sound like that is the case at all. So I'll just reiterate an earlier part of my answer: sounds like you like it, and I think you should continue liking it! There is not nearly enough fun and play in our day-to-day lives, so grab as much of it as you can, as guilt-free as you possibly can. Ok?

Auntie

Dear Auntie,

I have a very specific fetish. How do I make sure that people I date know that I like them for themselves and not only because they fit my type?

Hey there, my nibling,

I'm super attracted to smart people. An intellecta-sexual if you will. So my attraction to someone does begin with them fitting my type. That's ok. If you read the rest of this book, you've seen as much evidence as I could shove in about how normal it is to like what you like. We don't get super judgey when someone says they love redheads, or big boobs, or tall, athletic men or whatever. So liking someone because of your fetish is the same thing.

The thing you need to do is embrace that you don't like them *exclusively* because they fit your type. That was your initial pants-attraction moment, but they are also great in so many other ways. Lean into the emotional honesty of that. Compliment the other things about them that you adore, not just the things involving your fetish.

For example, say you have a foot fetish. Demonstrating attention and affection toward your partner's recent pedicure is totally fine. But also make sure you mention how grateful you are that they dropped off your lunch at your work. That they're kind to your nutty family. That they are always down for a B-movie watch party. Because a shitty human with great feet might be fun for a little while, but it's not a sustaining feature.

Auntie

Dear Auntie,

I'm a straight female and sometimes I like to watch porn with men fucking each other and sometimes I like to watch porn with women fucking each other. It seems very confusing to me, is there a word for someone who is straight who enjoys watching gay and lesbian porn? I used to be a dancer, so maybe it has something to do with that. I don't know, I've shared this info and people say it's normal . . . thank you.

Hey there, my niece!

Your people who tell you "girl, super normal" are super right. And great and supportive friends, by the way. But here is some data to back you up. Back in 2015, Pornhub published their finding that a solid third of their viewers of gay male porn were straight women. Sexuality researcher Lucy Neville was fascinated by this, and she surveyed and interviewed 500 straight women and published a book of her findings called *Girls Who Like Boys Who Like Boys*. And it turns out there are tons of reasons why this is the case.

Some people feel that queer porn is more ethical because it takes out the exploitive dynamics that are present way too fucking often in straight porn. There is more equity in the pleasure being experienced, even in the porn that is rougher. Others report that they like that it is more versatile, and surprising and creative and innovative—not just kiss kiss, lick lick, now PENETRATION AND ORGASM.

Meh. Boring.

You mentioned being a dancer, so you might be drawn to the aesthetics of bodies. Other women gave a similar reason for liking queer porn: the focus on how bodies are shown tends to be different, including how we show people's faces when they're experiencing pleasure.

The gay male porn specifically allows women to fantasize about what it would be like to have sex as a man . . . not because they are secretly transmasc (at least most of the time) but because it is fun to play with the idea of being someone other than yourself. Or the idea of being with someone who is different from your real-life partner(s), in the case of women who have sex with women.

And what about lesbian porn? The research in that area is incredibly similar. The number one porn-related search term by women, both on Pornhub (according to a 2019 report, this time) and in general, is "lesbian." There is far more centering of vaginal and clitoral pleasure in lesbian porn, as well as story lines that make it easier to visualize ourselves in the situations being portrayed.

And lastly, either way, it's fun and subversive to like something just because it wasn't made specifically for you. Sometimes it's just fun to be a little naughty, right?

All this is to say, you don't need to overthink your own identity because you like queer porn. It's a way of engaging with our rich inner world, without doing things we aren't actually interested in doing. Violent crime podcasts are also seriously popular, right? I just checked to see what the top 10 podcasts were on my Apple Podcasts app. Half of them were about violent crime. That doesn't mean millions of people are violent criminals, it's just another indication that we are always interested in exploring different facets of humanity.

Auntie

Dear Auntie,

*Is it normal to sometimes prefer just watching porn and
getting done with it rather than doing the whole sex
thing? I'm tired and I want to see my boyfriend orgasm,
and both of us jerking off is frankly the easiest thing. I
worry that it might make our sex lazy.*

Dear nibling,

Mutual masturbation (porn-enhanced, in your case) lets you
tend to your own needs efficiently, focus on your own pleasure
specifically, and still enjoy some connection with your partner. Even
if that was the entirety of y'all's shared sex lives, if you are both super
happy with the arrangements? Not every meal has to be a fancy,
eight-course affair. You're allowed to have a grab-and-go and find
it also fucking delicious. Y'all deserve the sex lives that suit you
best. And everyone can go fuck themselves . . . because (dad joke
incoming) y'all already are.

Auntie

Dear Auntie,

*My boyfriend really enjoys being flogged and whipped. I
really want to do this for him, but it breaks my heart to
hurt him. Can you help me reframe this in a way that I
can see the excitement and fun he is getting from it?*

Dear nibling,

I love you so much for loving your boyfriend so much. If you
find pain to be . . . well, painful . . . wrapping your head around him
having a different experience of pain will be difficult. Most people
wouldn't bother trying, but you really want to step into his worldview

to show up for him in the ways he desires. You're amazing for that, so thank you!

Here's the tea. Pain and pleasure exist in the same parts of the brain. We know this because a bunch of fancy-pants radiology professors at Harvard were frustrated with the medical field's inability to treat chronic pain well and wanted to see what was going on in the brain when people experience pain. And they found out that the brain lights up the way it does for money, food, and sex. This is also why people like hella spicy foods, actually. It's sorta sexual. A little bit of pain helps us release our natural analgesics so we feel grounded and relaxed and embodied and focused. This makes sense in light of some other research that demonstrates that BDSM may be the most mindful kind of sex we can have. So when he says it feels good, is relaxing, etc. . . . it's totally true. He's feeling embodied and engaged and his brain and body are super happy with the experience.

So talk to him about limits, and aftercare, and all that other important stuff so you can have some safeties to lean into since this is new for you. But you can trust what he is telling you about his experiences, the science backs him up.

Auntie

Dear Auntie Faith,

How would you recommend someone explore their kink in a safe way so that any vanilla part of their life is unaffected? For instance, if someone is afraid of being exposed or blackmailed by reaching out to others online, or of being threatened with exposure if they meet up with an individual or attend a group event?

Nibling,

Unfortunately, there isn't any such thing as complete safety. Even if you go to some costumed event (which may be a good idea for you, actually), if you have a birthmark shaped like Alaska that someone recognizes? You still may get popped.

That being said, I know lots of people with very public lives that safely kink. You want to be involved in spaces where privacy is explicated and protected to all extents possible. If you are looking for events and meet-ups, consider looking for ones where you have to reach out to the organizers to get information to attend. Anything publicly posted may attract problematic individuals. Many events are held at private residences instead of clubs for just that reason. I've taught at several of them over the years, actually. They have never felt weird or unsafe to me; in fact, I found them to feel safer and the people to be very polite and kind because the coordinators had curated who was going to be there.

This is a place where having an account on FetLife (without your pic or identifying info) can help you start making some connections. You can also ask at your local sex toy stores. I know other people who travel for their sexyfuntimes. Some go to a different city if they want to visit a club, and others go to events outside of the country . . . like swingers events at Caribbean resorts or whatever.

If you are super famous and fancy, having partners sign a non-disclosure agreement may already be a part of your life and would also apply here. Even if you aren't famous and fancy, NDAs make a solid deterrent for many people, though they aren't super enforceable in court (and actually are straight-up illegal to invoke in sexual harassment cases starting in 2023). I included one in the appendix of this book based just on this question, so check that out and see if it's helpful.

And again, consider attending masked events. Just cover all weird birthmarks and tattoos with some Dermablend first.

Auntie

Dear Auntie,

Why do I love sensory deprivation during impact play?

Hi, nibling!

While YMMV, the general research behind sensory deprivation tells us that people really dig it for a couple of reasons that may align with your experience. The general, smaller idea relates to all the reasons we like BDSM in general. Safely playing with power, etc. But there is also a bigger idea behind sensory deprivation.

The idea is that when certain senses go offline, or are muffled, it heightens our other senses. People who have lost their vision or hearing because of illness or accident (versus being born without it) also consistently report stronger experiences of their other senses. My guess is that this is also an evolutionary feature. Your body is trying to make sense of the world and your safety within it and will try to take in further, say, smell information when sight isn't available. In your case, touch becomes heightened, and wanted touch feels ahhhhh-mayyyyyy-zzzzzzzing, because you aren't having to filter out other sensory data in order to focus on it.

So you could really lean into that, adding different textural experiences like feathers or suede or whatever. And maybe explore temperature play if you haven't already. Try cold, carbonated soda followed by warm mint tea, which offers different temperatures plus some bonus tingles. Keep enjoying yourself, your partner(s), and your body . . . we're supposed to!

Auntie

Dear Auntie,

Why do I feel free when I'm in bondage?

Hi there, my nibling,

Of course there isn't likely one singular reason. And of course your reasons may not be listed below, but research around this topic gives us a couple possible ideas. While in bondage, you aren't actually disempowered. In fact (as mentioned elsewhere in this book), you are the one who has all of the power. You feel safe, and cared for, and can relax into the experience rather than having to make things happen for yourself.

My personal and professional experiences (this is me saying that this is not an evidence-based-practice statement, but instead a practice-based-evidence one) are that the strongest, most powerful, epic boss people are the ones that most like being submissive in these dynamics. It's a lovely break from the rest of their lives. A dom friend of mine remarked some years ago that this is what makes the dynamic so hot for him. Some powerful woman who could crush him like a bug in the business world trusts him to hold space for her to enjoy this experience? Incredibly sexy. We love a dom who loves and respects strong partners, amiright?

There is also the possibility that it's even more physiological than that. Subspace (that float-y, relaxed feeling that submissives experience during BDSM play) can feel trancelike, or dissociative-adjacent. Which means we are engaging with some dorsal vagal tone. And THAT means we are releasing dopamine, endorphins, cholecystokinin, catecholamines, substance P, and angiotensin II. And all that shit feels really good in and of itself.

And without a prescription. Look at you, hacking the system!

Auntie

Dear Auntie,

I'm interested in BDSM but my husband is not. How would you recommend I have the conversation with him about my desire? And is there a way to safely and respectfully explore this on my own?

Dear nibling,

I had a conversation about this recently, which ended with the person I was talking to saying that I should make a conversation deck just for this topic. So I did, and that might be something you want to play with. But self-promotion aside, the fact that this question has come up regularly for me means this is a huge need that society has not been great at addressing pragmatically. Earlier in this book I talked about the yes/no/maybe checklists that offer different options, which may be a good starting point to y'alls conversation, as well. And those don't require you to give me any more of your money.

Also offer him ways to dip his toes in the water, so to speak, without throwing him in the deep end. Ask him if he would be willing to go to a munch, since it is a meet-and-greet and no sexytimes will be happening. See if he is interested in going to a show that features elements of BDSM. Some burlesque performers, for example, play with their performances in this way. There are also BDSM fashion shows showcasing all of the associated accoutrements, which may be a safe starting point. Any media that involves BDSM and presents it in an erotic way might also be a good start. Porn is awesome, but it doesn't have to be porn. Earlier in this book, I suggested the movie *Secretary* as another example. Photographs and drawings may feel safer yet. Don't dump all of this on him, but tell him you were kinda wanting to check it out and ask if he would be willing to explore with you.

If anything around BDSM is just a hard-limit no-no for him, then have the honest conversation about your interest in the topic and negotiate your relationship boundaries around it. If y'all already have open borders around some activities (watching porn, going to clubs, whatever), then let him know you are going to explore for yourself, but following those parameters. If new parameters need to be discussed, do so concretely and specifically. As in "I'm going to this kink show, and I'd like to go back to the spanking room and get spanked. I don't plan on having any connection with anyone there beyond that interaction, but it is still different enough from our regular interactions that I'd like for us to talk about it and make that decision together."

Auntie

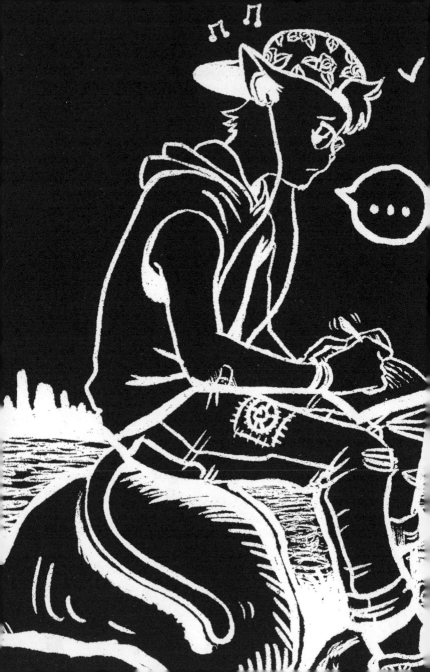

KINK-CLUSION

I would first of all just like to say how much I hate writing conclusions to my books, and continue to put it off until we are well into edits and I'm getting very patient reminders that it is time to do so. And I also hate it because I have never gotten any better at it over the years. Maybe because I don't like the idea of a conclusion in general (I JUST CAN'T QUIT YOU!), but probably because I still have flashbacks to 10th-grade English, where my teacher was obsessed with us crafting these perfect five-paragraph essays with a concluding paragraph that recapped everything we'd said. And I am a cranky Gen Xer who hasn't gotten any better at doing what I am told to do.

While covering everything there is to know about kink would be impossible, even if I was filling a multi-volume encyclopedia, I do hope (see! I am concluding!) that this was a helpful introduction to the topics that people have expressed the most interest in and asked me the most questions about. They are the topics that come up most often not just in my practice, but also in those of my fellow sex-positive clinical colleagues. And I hope you enjoyed nerding out over the science of sexuality and kink as much as I did.

Most importantly, though, I hope this book has helped you understand and begin to overcome any shame you might have felt for liking what you like. I mean, even if we didn't have any science behind these topics, the answer would be "you are literally hurting no one . . . except consensually with your nice purple flogger . . . so continue to enjoy yourself." But in truth, we do have research. Research that shows, over and over again, that there is literally no evidence that kinky practices are harmful. And that in fact, the evidence suggests that these practices have evolutionary reasons for existing and can be incredibly healing.

And if being Team Science means you also get to enjoy your sexytimes even more? That's (literally) fucking awesome.

Go forth, you little pervert.

RESOURCES

*I*f this book has piqued your interest in learning more about kink and human sexuality in general, check out the recs below for some further reading on these topics. I've also included some legal resources and some resources for clinicians.

And here's a note on book publishers: You will find that certain publishers specialize more in kink-forward books (both fiction and nonfiction) than others. One of the biggest names in nonfiction kink guides, Greenery Press, ceased publishing new titles in 2019, though many of their books are still easy to find. Another big name, Cleis Press, is still in operation and publishes great stuff. As does the publisher that put out this book . . . Microcosm Publishing. When I find a book I like, I look at who published it and what else they publish. I hope you'll do the same so you can continue to build knowledge in this area, if you are into that. It's exactly how I ended up publishing with Microcosm. I thought they published the coolest shit, and I wanted to be on that roster, and they eventually agreed!

Evolutionary Psychology of Sex
Why Is the Penis Shaped Like That? And Other Reflections on Being Human Jesse Bering

Perv: The Sexual Deviant in All of Us Jesse Bering

Sex-Positive Reading List

Pleasure Activism: The Politics of Feeling Good adrienne maree brown

Insatiable Wives: Women Who Stray and the Men Who Love Them David Ley

Ethical Porn for Dicks: A Man's Guide to Responsible Viewing Pleasure David Ley

The Myth of Sex Addiction David Ley

SM 101: A Realistic Introduction Jay Wiseman

The Big Book for Littles: Tips & Tricks for Age Players & Their Partners Penny Barber

Who's Been Sleeping in Your Head: The Secret World of Sexual Fantasies Brett Kahr

Sex Outside the Lines: Authentic Sexuality in a Sexually Dysfunctional Culture Chris Donaghue

Rebel Love: Break the Rules, Destroy Toxic Habits, and Have the Best Sex of Your Life Chris Donaghue and Amber Rose

Sexual Intelligence: What We Really Want from Sex—and How to Get It Marty Klein

Tell Me What You Want: The Science of Sexual Desire and How It Can Help You Improve Your Sex Life Justin J. Lehmiller

Come As You Are: Revised and Updated: The Surprising New Science That Will Transform Your Sex Life (**book and workbook**) Emily Nagoski

Mating in Captivity: Unlocking Erotic Intelligence Esther Perel

Unfuck Your Intimacy: Using Science for Better Relationships, Sex, and Dating Dr. Faith G. Harper

Unfuck Your Blow Jobs: How to Give and Receive Glorious Head Dr. Faith G. Harper

Unfuck Your Cunnilingus: How to Give and Receive Tongue-Twisting Oral Sex Dr. Faith G. Harper

Unfuck Your Sex Toys: Make Your Own DIY Tools and MacGyver Your Sexytimes Dr. Faith G. Harper

Sexing Yourself: Masturbation for Your Own Pleasure (**zine**) Dr. Faith G. Harper

Consent and Boundaries

The Art of Receiving and Giving: The Wheel of Consent Betty Martin and Robyn Dalzen

Empowered Boundaries: Speaking Truth, Setting Boundaries, and Inspiring Social Change Cristien Storm

Set Boundaries, Find Peace: A Guide to Reclaiming Yourself Nedra Glover Tawwab

Unfuck Your Boundaries: Build Better Relationships through Consent, Communication, and Expressing Your Needs (**book and workbook**) Dr. Faith G. Harper

Boundaries Conversation Deck: What Would You Do? (**card deck**) Dr. Faith G. Harper

Unfuck Your Consent: A History and How-To for Claiming Your Sexual Autonomy, Personal Boundaries, and Political Freedoms (zine) Dr. Faith G. Harper

Resources for Legal Support

National Coalition for Sexual Freedom ncsfreedom.org

Stop FOSTA/SESTA stopsesta.org

"DSM-5 and Paraphilic Disorders" (article in the *Journal of the American Academy of Psychiatry and the Law*) PMID: 24986346 Michael B. First

Resources for Clinicians and Coaches

Problem Sexual Behavior Certification Program— Sexual Health Alliance sexualhealthalliance.com/problem-sexual-behavior

Sexual Health Training (Out of Control Sexual Behavior Certification Program) theharveyinstitute.com

A Strength-Based Approach to Treating Out of Control Sexual Behavior (OCSB) drtammynelson.com

Declaration of Sexual Rights worldsexualhealth.net

Working Definitions after WHO Technical Consultation on Sexual Health worldsexualhealth.net

Kink Education Code of Conduct thekecc.org

Clinical Practice Guidelines for Working with People with Kink Interests kinkguidelines.com

Elemental Kink Readiness to Advanced Kink Proficiencies for Medical and Mental Health Providers kinkguidelines.com

APPENDIX: CONTRACT TEMPLATES

*B*oth of these sample contracts are available for educational purposes only. Because I obviously am not a lawyer and should not be trusted as legal counsel on such matters. However, I did have my lawyer bestie[9] review the sample contracts I found on the National Coalition for Sexual Freedom website (the consent contract) and PandaDoc (the relationship NDA) and fix a few things that were unclear on our behalves. So hopefully they will be a good starting point for you, too!

Sample Consent Contract

Since our contemporary conversation around consent started within the kink community, let's look at one of the more formal consent tools that has come from the aforementioned community. Some people may snicker at the idea, but a written consent contract doesn't exist for the purpose of earning extra-woke brownie points. They make legal sense for BDSM play, but even more so . . . they create a foundation and structure for a conversation about active, continuous consent. Which is my polite way of saying that even a contract can be revoked at any time. And that's not woke-ness . . . that's badass, thoughtful adulting.

---

9 Chase Jones, who practices family law and advocacy law in Texas and is clearly cool enough to consult with on a kink book if you ever need a rockstar attorney (chasejoneslaw.com).

I, _____, hereby declare under penalty of perjury that I am over 18 years old and am not under the influence of intoxicants or medications that inhibit my ability to affirm consent.

I further declare that this agreement is of my own free will and that neither I nor anyone near or dear to me has been threatened with negative consequences if I chose not to enter into this contract.

Both parties agree that this is a private agreement not to be disclosed to third parties except in case of accusation of sexual misconduct by an agreeing party.

If an agreeing party shows or makes public this agreement without accusation of sexual misconduct, it is agreed that they will be liable for damages for invasion of privacy.

By initialing, _____ I agree to engage in all or some of the following consensual acts:

With the following individual(s):

Safer sex methods that I want utilized during these acts include:

At this time I do not intend to change my mind before the sex act or acts are over. However, if I do, it is further understood that when I say the words _____ or make the signal (hand gesture, etc.) _____, all involved parties/partners agree to STOP INSTANTLY!

Signed:_____ Date:_____

Signed:_____ Date:_____

Disclaimer: This sample contract does not constitute legal advice and is provided for educational purposes only. Check with legal counsel before entering into any agreement.

Relationship Non-Disclosure Agreement Template

This template, based on a free one from PandaDoc (you can search for it and find it there super easily), is here to serve as an example of a relationship NDA. Do keep in mind that because NDAs have been weaponized by abusers in the past, the Speak Out Act (signed into law on December 7, 2022) states:

> No nondisclosure clause or nondisparagement clause agreed to before the dispute arises shall be judicially enforceable in instances in which conduct is alleged to have violated Federal, Tribal, or State law.

The idea is that NDAs cannot be used in cases of abuse and assault. This is true even if the NDA was signed before the law took effect. Additionally, the courts don't always uphold them because of their shady history. They are, however, a possible way of maintaining the privacy of consenting kinky sexyfuntimes, or at least making others hesitate before outing you. Especially if you have a level of community standing that could be impacted by your extracurriculars.

Prepared for:

[Party A.FirstName]

[Party A.LastName]

Created by:

[Party B.FirstName]

[Party B.LastName]

I. The Parties

This Mutual Relationship Non-Disclosure Agreement, hereinafter called "Relationship Agreement," effective as of (Date), hereinafter referred to as "Effective Date," is between the following two parties, hereinafter referred to as "Parties" or "Couple":

Party A: Described as 1 part of the Couple known as

[Party A.FirstName]

[Party A.LastName] ("Party A") who currently lives at

[Party A.StreetAddress],

[Party A.City],

[Party A.State],

[Party A.PostalCode] with a mailing address of

[Party A.StreetAddress],

[Party A.City],

[Party A.State],

[Party A.PostalCode]

AND

Party B: Described as 1 part of the Couple known as

[Party B.FirstName]

[Party B.LastName] ("Party B") who currently lives at

[Party B.StreetAddress],

[Party B.City],

[Party B.State],

[Party B.PostalCode] with a mailing address of

[Party B.StreetAddress],

[Party B.City],

[Party B.State],

[Party B.PostalCode].

II. *Confidential Information*

The phrase "Confidential Information" includes, but isn't limited to, details about the Couple's sex life, arguments (that don't involve abusive speech or become physical), extended family-related problems, finances, disappointments, insecurities, habits or experiences or addictions that were expressed as embarrassing, infidelity, opinions discussed in confidence, past relationship failures and/or anything else both Parties deemed private.

All Confidential Information must remain private regardless of how the included information was delivered. Text messages, notes, speech, emails, and private social media correspondence are all considered proper communication channels that are subject to Section II.

III. *Non-Disclosure*

The couple agrees that they shall have an obligation to

Hold all written Confidential Information in the strictest of confidence,

Never use any Confidential Information to defame the other Party,

Never use any Confidential Information for personal gain,

Not disclose what Confidential Information is or isn't available to a third party,

Take the steps necessary to ensure Confidential Information is guarded.

Section III shall remain and continue after the termination or expiration of the relationship between the two Parties and bind the Couple regardless of when, how, or why both Parties "broke up."

IV. Exceptions to Section II
The Couple agrees that the following topics are not restricted:

Any information that was made public on the individual whims of one of the Parties (for example, information Party A posted to their own social media account or topics Party A discussed on a live broadcast freely without coercion are considered public knowledge).

Any information that came to be public domain through no fault of the Parties (for example, a third party made something Party B told them in confidence public).

Any information that was known by Party A or Party B before confidence was communicated or if confidence wasn't directly communicated firstly but later corrected.

Any information that was independently found by the Couple without it being communicated to them by Party A or Party B in the past, present, or future.

Any information provided by a court, government body, or law enforcement.

Any information that Party A or Party B provided written or verbal notice for approval.

Any information that could be considered illegal, a threat of harm, or an emergency.

Any information that could suggest or provide evidence of physical, sexual, or emotional abuse or neglect of any other third party or one or more members of the Couple.

V. *Use of Confidential Information*

All Confidential Information outlined in Section II shall only be discussed between the Couple unless deemed otherwise. Confidential Information may be discussed with a non-biased third party that must maintain confidentiality as a part of their profession or services (for example, a couples therapist or psychologist).

VI. *Notice of Disclosure*

Parties must give at least [length of time in hours/days/weeks] notice before discussing Confidential Information with anyone unless the person(s) in question are a non-biased third-party mental health doctor or physician, a governing body, or a legal entity.

Parties are responsible for notifying the other Party of the circumstances surrounding the request for information unless doing so violates applicable laws or statutes.

Parties cannot disclose information to a third party and ask for permission at a later date. Even if permission is granted after the fact, Parties still violate the Relationship Agreement.

VII. Term

This Relationship Agreement will remain in effect for perpetuity.

VIII. Return of Confidential Information

If the Confidential Information in question has a physical component, it must be returned within [length of time in hours/ days/weeks] after the Couple declares their separation. Both Parties will return all equipment, documents, materials, records, or anything else that includes the Confidential Information and not make copies.

IX. Reason for Covenant

This covenant or legal agreement is agreed by both Parties as necessary to protect the goodwill and reputation of Party A and Party B. Each party consents to this agreement after having a sufficient opportunity to consult with a licensed attorney of their choice regarding the legal rights and consequences of this agreement.

X. Reparations and Enforcement

Should one or more Parties break the Relationship Agreement, they acknowledge that they would cause irreparable harm in which equitable damages and relief can be sought. The violated party is and henceforth entitled to all remedies available from the law. If any of the information in this Relationship Agreement is considered unenforceable, all other remaining provisions shall not be affected, and the rights of the Parties shall be enforced.

XI. Assignment and Authority

This Relationship Agreement cannot be assigned to another party or edited by the Couple unless both Party A and Party B provide written consent.

Each Party will represent and adhere to the original written document and acknowledge that the signed copy of this Relationship Agreement holds full authority and power for perpetuity.

XII. Execution

IN WITNESS WHEREOF, the Couple agrees that this Relationship Agreement will come into effect on

Signature _____

Date _____

[Party A.FirstName]

[Party A.LastName]

[Party A.Company]

Signature _____

Date _____

[Party B.FirstName]

[Party B.LastName]

[Party B.Company]

REFERENCES

117th Congress (2021–2022): Speak out act. (n.d.). congress.gov/bill/117th-congress/senate-bill/4524/text

Admin, B. (2023, April 22). The end of a police roundtable makes some Portland kinksters nervous. National Coalition for Sexual Freedom. ncsfreedom.org/2023/04/22/the-end-of-a-police-roundtable-makes-some-portland-kinksters-nervous/

Banmen, J. (2002). The Satir model: Yesterday and today. *Contemporary Family Therapy*, 24(1), 7–22.

Basson, R. (2005). Women's sexual dysfunction: Revised and expanded definitions. *CMAJ: Canadian Medical Association journal = journal de l'Association medicale canadienne*. 172. 1327–33. 10.1503/cmaj.1020174.

Baur, E., Forsman, M., Santtila, P., Johansson, A., Sandnabba, K., & Långström, N. (2016). Paraphilic sexual interests and sexually coercive behavior: A population-based twin study. *Archives of Sexual Behavior*, 45(5), 1163–1172. doi.org/10.1007/s10508-015-0674-2

Bering, J. (2015). *Perv*. Random House UK.

Bering, J. (2013). *Why is the penis shaped like that?* Transworld Publishers Ltd.

Blunt, D., & Wolf, A. Erased: The impact of FOSTA-SESTA and the removal of Backpage on sex workers. *Anti-Trafficking Review*, issue 14, 2020, 117–121, doi.org/10.14197/atr.201220148

Berman, L., Berman, J., Miles, M., Pollets, D., & Powell, J. A. (2003). Genital self-image as a component of sexual health: Relationship between genital self-image, female sexual function, and quality of life measures. *Journal of Sex & Marital Therapy*, 29 Suppl 1, 11–21. doi.org/10.1080/713847124

Brice, R. (2019, August 1). U up? How does HRT affect your sex and libido? Healthline. Retrieved October 14, 2021, from healthline.com/health/healthy-sex/hrt-sexuality-libido#4.

Calabrò, R. S., Cacciola, A., Bruschetta, D., Milardi, D., Quattrini, F., Sciarrone, F., la Rosa, G., Bramanti, P., & Anastasi, G. (2019). Neuroanatomy and function of human sexual behavior: A neglected or unknown issue? *Brain and Behavior*, 9(12), e01389. doi.org/10.1002/brb3.1389

Carrellas, B., & Sprinkle, A. (2017). *Urban tantra: Sacred sex for the twenty-first century*. Ten Speed Press.

Castellini, G., Rellini, A. H., Appignanesi, C., Pinucci, I., Fattorini, M., Grano, E., Fisher, A. D., Cassioli, E., Lelli, L., Maggi, M., & Ricca, V. (2018). Deviance or normalcy? The relationship among paraphilic thoughts and behaviors, hypersexuality, and psychopathology in a sample of university students. *The Journal of Sexual Medicine*, 15(9), 1322–1335. doi.org/10.1016/j.jsxm.2018.07.015

Center for Women's Health. OHSU. (n.d.). Retrieved October 14, 2021, from ohsu.edu/womens-health/benefits-healthy-sex-life.

Centers for Disease Control and Prevention. (2020, September 16). *Disability and health overview.* Centers for Disease Control and Prevention. Retrieved November 16, 2021, from cdc.gov/ncbddd/disabilityandhealth/disability.html.

Centers for Disease Control and Prevention. (2020, September 16). *Disability impacts all of us infographic.* Centers for Disease Control and Prevention. Retrieved November 16, 2021, from cdc.gov/ncbddd/disabilityandhealth/infographic-disability-impacts-all.html#:%7E:text=61%E2%80%8Amillion%E2%80%8Aadults%E2%80%8Ain%E2%80%8Athe%2Chave%E2%80%8Asome%E2%80%8Atype%E2%80%8Aof%E2%80%8Adisability.

Chen, A. (2020, September 9). What brain scans tell us about sex. The Maudern. Retrieved October 14, 2021, from getmaude.com/blogs/themaudern/on-what-brain-scans-can-tell-us-about-sex.

Chivers, M. L., & Bailey, J. M. (2005). A sex difference in features that elicit genital response. *Biological Psychology, 70*(2), 115–120. doi.org/10.1016/j.biopsycho.2004.12.002

Chivers, M.L. The specificity of women's sexual response and its relationship with sexual orientations: A review and ten hypotheses. *Archives of Sexual Behavior 46,* 1161–1179 (2017). doi.org/10.1007/s10508-016-0897-x

Cleveland Clinic (2021). Sexual response cycle: What it is, phases. Cleveland Clinic. my.clevelandclinic.org/health/articles/9119-sexual-response-cycle

Clews, C. (2014, April 7). 1987. Politics: Operation spanner. Gay in the 80s. gayinthe80s.com/2014/04/1987-politics-operation-spanner/

Cromie, W. J. (2002, January 31). Pleasure, pain activate same part of brain. *Harvard Gazette*. news.harvard.edu/gazette/story/2002/01/pleasure-pain-activate-same-part-of-brain/

Diamond, M. (2009). Pornography, public acceptance and sex related crime: A review. *International Journal of Law and Psychiatry*, 32(5), 304–314. doi.org/10.1016/j.ijlp.2009.06.004

Discipline (n.). Etymology. (n.d.). etymonline.com/word/discipline#:~:text=discipline%20(v.),train%22%20is%20from%20late%2014c.

Discipline. Urban Dictionary. (n.d.). urbandictionary.com/define.php?term=discipline

Do people in the Pokemon world have fetishes for Pokemon? Quora. (n.d.). quora.com/Do-people-in-the-Pokemon-world-have-fetishes-for-Pokemon

Dumais, E., (2021a, August 9). A guide to sensory deprivation. The Maudern. getmaude.com/blogs/themaudern/blindfold-sex#:~:text=Certainly%20an%20apt%20question%E2%80%94but,sensory%20information%20to%20heighten%20others.

Edenfield, A. C. (2019, March 10). Queering consent: Design and sexual consent messaging. ACM SIGDOC. sigdoc.acm.org/cdq/queering-consent-design-and-sexual-consent-messaging/

Ellis, A. (1964). Nymphomania: A study of the oversexed woman. Gilbert Press.

Emery, L. R. (2016, September 29). BDSM may be the most mindful type of sex, study finds. Bustle. bustle.com/articles/186777-bdsm-may-be-the-most-mindful-type-of-sex-study-finds

Exploring the benefits of sensory deprivation sexual experiences. Allo Health. (2023, July 1). allohealth.care/healthfeed/sex-education/sensory-deprivation-sexual

Free relationship non-disclosure agreement template—get 2023 sample. PandaDoc. (2023, May 7). pandadoc.com/relationship-non-disclosure-agreement-template/

Giannini, A.J., Colapietro, G., Slaby, A.E., Melemis, S.M. & Bowman, RK (1998). Sexualization of the female foot as a response to sexually transmitted epidemics: A preliminary study. *Psychological Reports*, 83, 491-498.

Haber, R. (2002). Virginia Satir: An integrated, humanistic approach. *Contemporary Family Therapy*, 24(1), 23–34.

Haidt, J. The emotional dog and its rational tail: A social intuitionist approach to moral judgment. *Psychological Review*, 2001, 108(4), 814–834. doi.org/10.1037/0033-295X.108.4.814

Haidt, J., Björklund F., & Murphy S. (2000). *Moral dumbfounding: When intuition finds no reason.* University of Virginia Unpublished Manuscript.

Haidt, J., Björklund, F., & Sinnott-Armstrong, W. Social intuitionists answer six questions about moral psychology. *Moral psychology volume 2: The cognitive science of morality: Intuition and diversity*, 2008, LondonMIT, 181–217.

Herbenick, D., et al. Sexual diversity in the United States: Results from a nationally representative probability sample of adult men and women. PLoS One. July 20, 2017. doi.org/10.1371/journal.pone.0181198.

Holvoet, L., et al. (2017). Fifty shades of Belgian gray: The prevalence of BDSM-related fantasies and activities in the general population. *Journal of Sexual Medicine*, 14(9), 1152–1159. doi: 10.1016/j.jsxm.2017.07.003

Iovine, A. (2023, January 27). Kinktok is rife with misinformation. Here's why that's dangerous. Mashable. mashable.com/article/kinktok-tiktok-kink-community

Journalist, L. S. D. (2023, February 21). How many Americans prefer non-monogamy in relationships? YouGov. today. yougov.com/topics/society/articles-reports/2023/02/21/how-many-americans-prefer-nonmonogamy-relationship

Joyal, C. C., & Carpentier, J. (2017). The prevalence of paraphilic interests and behaviors in the general population: A provincial survey. *Journal of Sex Research*, 54(2), 161–171.

Kafka, M. P. (2010). Hypersexual disorder: A proposed diagnosis for DSM-V. *Archives of Sexual Behavior*, 39(2), 377–400. doi. org/10.1007/s10508-009-9574-7

Keene, L. C., & Davies, P. H. (1999). Drug-related erectile dysfunction. *Adverse Drug Reactions and Toxicological Reviews*, 18(1), 5–24.

Kessler, A., Sollie, S., Challacombe, B., Briggs, K., & Van Hemelrijck, M. (2019). The global prevalence of erectile dysfunction: A review. *BJU International*, 124(4), 587–599. doi. org/10.1111/bju.14813

Kinsey, A. C. (1998). *Sexual behavior in the human female*. Indiana University Press.

Kinsey, A. C., Pomeroy, W. B., & Martin, C. E. (1953). Sexual behavior in the human male. Saunders.

Knapp, H. (2006). Pornography - The secret history of civilisation [DVD]. United Kingdom; Koch Vision.

Leslie, R. A. (1985). The distributions of classical and putative neurotransmitters within somata and fibres of the dorsal vagal complex are reviewed. The occurrence within the dorsal medulla oblongata of receptors specific for some of these substances is examined. Neuroactive substances in the dorsal vagal complex of the medulla oblongata: Nucleus of the tractus solitarius, area postrema, and dorsal motor nucleus of the Vagus. *Neurochemistry International*. sciencedirect. com/science/article/abs/pii/0197018685901068

Let's discuss consensual non-consent, shall we? *Cosmopolitan*. (2022, September 13). cosmopolitan.com/sex-love/a41175223/consensual-non-consent/

Levy, M. S. (1998). A helpful way to conceptualize and understand reenactments. Journal of Psychotherapy Practice and Research, 7(3), 227–235.

Ley, D. J. (2011). Insatiable wives: Women who stray and the men who love them. Rowman & Littlefield.

Ley, D. J. (2014). The myth of sex addiction. Rowman & Littlefield.

Ley, D. J. (2016). Ethical porn for dicks: A man's guide to responsible viewing pleasure. Essay, ThreeL Media.

Ley, D. (n.d.). Criminal charges and consensual kink. *Psychology Today*. psychologytoday.com/us/blog/women-who-stray/202306/criminal-charges-and-consensual-kink

Lucas, J. (2023, April 19). After these people tried erotic hypnosis, they couldn't recognize themselves. BuzzFeed News. buzzfeednews.com/article/jessicalucas2/erotic-hypnosis-bambi-sleep

MacLeod, C.M. (2020). Zeigarnik and von Restorff: The memory effects and the stories behind them. *Memory & Cognition* 48, 1073–1088. doi.org/10.3758/s13421-020-01033-5

Mashable SEA. (2023, April 6). A beginner's guide to impact play. Mashable SEA. sea.mashable.com/life/23048/a-beginners-guide-to-impact-play

Mayo Foundation for Medical Education and Research. (2021, July 9). Viagra and other erectile dysfunction drugs: Understand how they work. Mayo Clinic. Retrieved October 13, 2021, from mayoclinic.org/diseases-conditions/erectile-dysfunction/in-depth/erectile-dysfunction/art-20047821.

MehaffyWeber. (2023, January 9). New federal law bans NDAs in sexual harassment cases. MehaffyWeber. mehaffyweber.com/news/federal-law-bans-ndas-in-sexual-harassment-cases/#:~:text=The%20law%20makes%20it%20illegal,when%20the%20NDA%20was%20dated.

Mehrotra, D. (2023, June 12). An anti-porn app put him in jail and his family under surveillance. Wired. wired.com/story/anti-porn-covenant-eyes-bond-revoked/

Mitrokostas, B. I. (n.d.). Here's what happens to your body and brain when you orgasm. ScienceAlert. Retrieved November 19, 2021, from sciencealert.com/here-s-what-happens-to-your-brain-when-you-orgasm.

Molen, L. V., Ronis, S. T., & Benoit, A. A. (2023). Paraphilic interests versus behaviors: Factors that distinguish individuals who act on paraphilic interests from individuals who refrain. *Sexual Abuse: A Journal of Research and Treatment, 35*(4), 403–427. doi.org/10.1177/10790632221108949

MP. (2021, July 20). Sex club etiquette. Respark. respark.co/blog/sex-club-etiquette/

Muise, A., & Impett, E. A. (2014). Good, giving, and game. *Social Psychological and Personality Science, 6*(2), 164–172. doi.org/10.1177/1948550614553641

Muise, A., & Impett, E. A. (2016). Applying theories of communal motivation to sexuality. *Social and Personality Psychology Compass*, 10(8), 455–467. doi.org/10.1111/spc3.12261

NBCUniversal News Group. (2018, July 25). When no one is looking, many women are watching gay porn. NBCNews. com. nbcnews.com/feature/nbc-out/when-no-one-looking-many-women-are-watching-gay-porn-n894266

Oosterhuis, H. (2012). Sexual modernity in the works of Richard von Krafft-Ebing and Albert Moll. *Medical History*, 56(2), 133–155. doi.org/10.1017/mdh.2011.30

PandaDoc (2022). Free relationship non-disclosure agreement template—get 2023 sample. PandaDoc. (2023, August 7). pandadoc.com/relationship-non-disclosure-agreement-template/

Paraphilic Disorders. *Diagnostic and Statistical Manual of Mental Disorders* (Fifth ed.). American Psychiatric Publishing. 2013. pp. 685–686.

Pornhub. (October 13, 2017). Girls who like boys who like boys. Pornhub Insights. pornhub.com/insights/girls-like-boys-who-like-boys

Post-traumatic stress, sexual trauma and dissociative . . . (n.d.). Retrieved October 21, 2021, from ojp.gov/pdffiles1/Photocopy/153416NCJRS.pdf.

Prause, N. (2022, November 11). Anti-porn has a problem with false conspiracy theories. Medium. medium.com/@nicole.

prause/anti-porn-has-a-problem-with-false-conspiracy-theories-fc7385154371

Prause, N., & Binnie, J. (2022). Reboot/NoFap participants erectile concerns predicted by anxiety and not mediated/moderated by pornography viewing. *Journal of Psychosexual Health*, 4(4), 252–254. doi:10.1177/26318318221116354

Reid, R. C. (2015). How should severity be determined for the DSM-5 proposed classification of Hypersexual Disorder? *Journal of Behavioral Addictions*, 4(4), 221–225. doi.org/10.1556/2006.4.2015.041

Ross, C., & Dodson, B. (2017). Betty Dodson bodysex basics. Betty A. Dodson Foundation.

Russell, T. (2011). *A renegade history of the United States*. Free Press.

Sawyer, C. (2022, November 16). "Ethical sex-ploration" and two other trends that Bumble predicts will shape our dating lives in 2023. screenshot-media.com/the-future/dating/bumbles-2023-dating-trends-forecast/

Sayles, C. (2002). Transformational change—based on the model of Virginia Satir. *Contemporary Family Therapy*, 24(1), 93–109.

Schnarch, D. M. (2009). *Passionate marriage: Love, sex and intimacy in emotionally committed relationships*. W.W. Norton & Co.

Shea, A. (2022, August 23). Your guide to ethical porn: What makes it different & where to find it. Mindbodygreen. mindbodygreen.com/articles/ethical-porn

Smith, G. (2021, July 28). A BDSM beginner's guide to subspace. Healthline. healthline.com/health/healthy-sex/subspace-bdsm

Studd, J., & Schwenkhagen, A. (2009). The historical response to female sexuality. *Maturitas*, 63(2), 107–111. doi.org/10.1016/j.maturitas.2009.02.015

Study shatters the myth that BDSM is linked to early-life trauma. Big Think. (2022, April 19). bigthink.com/neuropsych/bdsm-psychology-trauma/

Sussex Publishers. (n.d.). Hypersexuality (sex addiction). *Psychology Today*. psychologytoday.com/us/conditions/hypersexuality-sex-addiction#:~:text=%22Sexual%20addiction%22%20and%20hypersexuality%20are,distress%2C%20specialized%20counseling%20is%20available.

Ten Brink, S., Coppens, V., Huys, W., et al. (2021). The psychology of kink: A survey study into the relationships of trauma and attachment style with BDSM interests. *Sexuality Research and Social Policy* 18, 1–12. doi.org/10.1007/s13178-020-00438-w

The end of a police roundtable makes some Portland kinksters nervous. *Willamette Week*. (n.d.). wweek.com/news/2023/04/05/the-end-of-a-police-roundtable-makes-some-portland-kinksters-nervous/

Tung, L. (2020, July 10). Fosta-Sesta was supposed to thwart sex trafficking. Instead, it's sparked a movement. WHYY. whyy.org/segments/fosta-sesta-was-supposed-to-thwart-sex-trafficking-instead-its-sparked-a-movement/

U.S. National Library of Medicine. (n.d.). Drugs that may cause erection problems. *Medlineplus Medical Encyclopedia*. MedlinePlus. Retrieved October 13, 2021, from medlineplus. gov/ency/article/004024.htm.

Waite, L. J., Laumann, E. O., Das, A., & Schumm, L. P. (2009). Sexuality: Measures of partnerships, practices, attitudes, and problems in the National Social Life, Health, and Aging Study. The Journals of Gerontology. Series B, Psychological Sciences and Social Sciences, 64 (Suppl 1), i56–i66. doi. org/10.1093/geronb/gbp038

WebMD. (n.d.). BDSM sex: What does it mean? WebMD. webmd. com/sex/what-is-bdsm-sex

Weiss, S. (2022, December 5). Is your kink actually a fetish? Let's break it down. *Men's Health*. menshealth.com/sex-women/ a42005563/kink-vs-fetish/

What is a substance use disorder? (n.d.). American Psychiatric Association. Retrieved January 17, 2022, from psychiatry. org/patients-families/addiction/what-is-addiction

Whipple, B., & Komisaruk, B. R. (1985). Elevation of pain threshold by vaginal stimulation in women. *Pain*, 21(4), 357–367. doi.org/10.1016/0304-3959(85)90164-2

Wikimedia Foundation. (2023, August 6). Ageplay. Wikipedia. en.wikipedia.org/wiki/Ageplay

Wise, N. J., Frangos, E., & Komisaruk, B. R. (2017). Brain activity unique to orgasm in women: An FMRI analysis. *The Journal of Sexual Medicine*, 14(11), 1380–1391. doi.org/10.1016/j.jsxm.2017.08.014

Women's Health Editors (2023, April 27). Here's exactly why straight women often prefer lesbian porn, according to sex experts. *Women's Health*. womenshealthmag.com/sex-and-love/a19947774/straight-women-lesbian-porn/

Yetman, D. (2020, March 5). How common is erectile dysfunction? Stats, causes, and treatment. Healthline. Retrieved October 21, 2021, from healthline.com/health/how-common-is-ed#prevalence.

ABOUT THE AUTHOR

Faith G. Harper, LPC-S, ACS, ACN, is a badass, funny lady with a PhD. She's a licensed professional counselor, board supervisor, certified sexologist, and applied clinical nutritionist with a private practice and consulting business in San Antonio, TX. She has been an adjunct professor and a TEDx presenter, and proudly identifies as a woman of color and uppity intersectional feminist. She is the author of dozens of books.

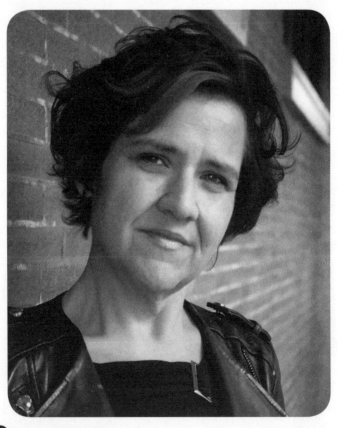

MORE BY DR. FAITH

Books
The Autism Partner Handbook (with Joe Biel and Elly Blue)
The Autism Relationships Handbook (with Joe Biel)
Befriend Your Brain
Coping Skills
How to Be Accountable (with Joe Biel)
This Is Your Brain on Depression
Unfuck Your Addiction
Unfuck Your Adulting
Unfuck Your Anger
Unfuck Your Anxiety
Unfuck Your Blow Jobs
Unfuck Your Body
Unfuck Your Boundaries
Unfuck Your Brain
Unfuck Your Cunnilingus
Unfuck Your Friendships
Unfuck Your Grief
Unfuck Your Intimacy
Unfuck Your Stress
Unfuck Your Worth
Unfuck Your Writing (with Joe Biel)
Woke Parenting (with Bonnie Scott)

Workbooks
Achieve Your Goals
The Autism Relationships Workbook (with Joe Biel)
How to Be Accountable Workbook (with Joe Biel)
Unfuck Your Anger Workbook
Unfuck Your Anxiety Workbook
Unfuck Your Body Workbook
Unfuck Your Boundaries Workbook
Unfuck Your Intimacy Workbook
Unfuck Your Worth Workbook

Unfuck Your Year
Zines
The Autism Handbook (with Joe Biel)
BDSM FAQ
Dating
Defriending
Detox Your Masculinity (with Aaron Sapp)
Emotional Freedom Technique
Getting Over It
How to Find a Therapist
How to Say No
Indigenous Noms
Relationshipping
The Revolution Won't Forget the Holidays
Self-Compassion
Sex Tools
Sexing Yourself
STI FAQ (with Aaron Sapp)
Surviving
This Is Your Brain on Addiction
This Is Your Brain on Grief
This Is Your Brain on PTSD
Unfuck Your Consent
Unfuck Your Forgiveness
Unfuck Your Mental Health Paradigm
Unfuck Your Sleep
Unfuck Your Work
Vision Boarding
Woke Parenting #1–6 (with Bonnie Scott)

Other
Boundaries Conversation Deck
Stress Coping Skills Deck
How Do You Feel Today? (poster)

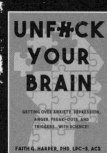

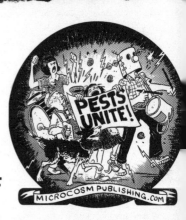
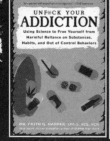
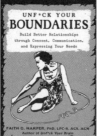
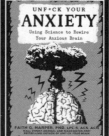
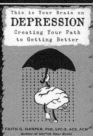